The FERTILITY HANDBOOK

A Guide to Getting Pregnant

C. Maud Doherty, M.D.

Melanie Morrissey Clark

Addicus Books
Omaha, Nebraska

An Addicus Nonfiction Book

ISBN 1-886039-55-0

Cover design by Peri Poloni

Illustrations by Jack Kusler

This book is not intended to serve as a substitute for a physician. Nor is it the authors' intent to give medical advice contrary to that of an attending physician's.

Library of Congress Cataloging-in-Publication Data

Doherty, C. Maud, 1958-
    The fertility handbook : a guide to getting pregnant / C. Maud Doherty, Melanie Morrissey Clark.
        p. cm.
"An Addicus Nonfiction Book."
Includes index.
    ISBN 1-886039-55-0 (alk. paper)
    1. Infertility—Popular works. I. Clark, Melanie Morrissey, 1966- II. Title.
    RC889 .D59 2002
    616.6'92—dc21

                                                2001006010

Addicus Books, Inc.
P.O. Box 45327
Omaha, Nebraska 68145
Web site: www.AddicusBooks.com

Printed in the United States of America
10 9 8 7 6 5 4 3 2 1

To my husband, Fred,
for giving me the strength to fight my infertility,
and to our three miracles, Cooper, Sophie, and Simon.
Melanie Morrissey Clark

To my children, Caity, Alex, and Grant,
my husband Mike,
my great staff, and all my patients.
C. Maud Doherty, M.D.

Contents

Acknowledgments

This book could not have been completed without the help of numerous individuals. We would like to thank Dr. Doherty's patients who shared their experiences, in turn providing guidance and emotional support to many others in need.

We would also like to thank Scott Sills, M.D. and Carolyn Kaplan, M.D., of Georgia Reproductive Specialists (IVF.com), for their editorial suggestions. We would also like to thank urologists Craig Niederberger, M.D., Chief of Andrology, University of Illinois, Chicago, and Jon Morton, M.D., Urology Center, Omaha, Nebraska, for their suggestions for the chapter on male factor infertility.

We would also like to thank Anne Steinhoff, Jill Bruckner Lynch, Amanda Duffy Randall, and Susan Adams for their help in providing feedback in the early stages of the manuscript.

Introduction

The realization that childbearing would not be easy for me was slow in coming, but when it finally arrived, it knocked me to my knees and left me breathless with indignation. Years later, I can still recall the mind-numbing fear I felt as I struggled with the thought that I may be infertile. Those feelings were often triggered by something as innocuous as a television advertisement for disposable diapers. I'd see the roly-poly babies laughing and crawling, and I'd think, I'll never have that...I'll never have a baby. My breath would shorten, my stomach would feel queasy and I would start to perspire. It would pass within a few minutes, and I would try to talk myself back into a more optimistic state of mind. This scene replayed itself many times during the four years it took me to get pregnant and carry a pregnancy to viability. It may sound familiar, or perhaps you have your own version of the story. We all do.

My Story

My journey through infertility began in 1993, with my first miscarriage at 12 weeks gestation. It had taken my husband, Fred, and me just five months to achieve a pregnancy, but the joy was short-lived. At my first doctor's appointment, we discovered the fetus had stopped growing. I tearfully scheduled the D&C (dilation and curettage) and went home to tell my family. Although my heart was heavy, I was confident that, at just 27 years old, I had experienced nothing more than the first-pregnancy loss common in many women. But I was wrong.

Two months later, I was pregnant again. This time the bleeding began just a few weeks after the pregnancy test, and we grieved once more. With this second loss came a creeping suspicion that something was wrong.

The next year of trying in vain to conceive forced me to face the facts, and I sought the help of a fertility specialist. Because I had been pregnant twice, this physician didn't think it necessary to do many tests. A hysterosalpingography (HSG) test to make sure my tubes were clear and a prescription for Clomid was all she thought I needed. Four months later, I was pregnant. But at what should have been nine weeks gestation, an ultrasound showed the fetus measured only six weeks, and there was no heartbeat. I was inconsolable for weeks after the D&C. Then, I made an appointment with reproductive endocrinologist C. Maud Doherty, M.D., my co-author.

Discovering the Problem

Dr. Doherty scheduled laparoscopic surgery, which allowed her to look inside my pelvis and discover I had severe, or stage-four, endometriosis. When I saw pictures of the scar tissue covering my uterus, bladder and other organs, my heart sank. I'd read about endometriosis and knew my advanced disease would make it difficult for me to conceive and carry a pregnancy to term. Still, I refused to give up.

My Course of Treatment

Dr. Doherty was optimistic, and as part of my treatment prescribed injectable super-ovulation drugs. At first my husband and I tried to conceive on our own, but when that didn't work we immediately moved forward with in vitro fertilization.

Although expensive, we knew this procedure offered us the best chance of success, and after three years, we were weary of waiting. When the first IVF did not result in a pregnancy, we were stunned and heartbroken. We talked about adoption, and the toll the treatments were taking on me, both physically and emotionally. Then we decided to give IVF one more try.

Success At Last

This time the pregnancy test was overwhelmingly positive. I saved the message Dr. Doherty left on my answering machine. "Your test is positive—really positive. We're probably looking at two or three here. Call me when you get in." Of course, that was only the beginning. My eventful triplet pregnancy included bleeding, pre-term labor and 10 weeks of bed rest—six of which were spent in the hospital—and a premature delivery at just over 31 weeks gestation. Our babies were born March 25, 1997—four years after my first miscarriage.

I'm a Mother

Thankfully, Cooper, at 4 pounds, 6 ounces; Sophie, at 3 pounds, 2 ounces; and Simon, at 2 pounds, 7 ounces, were all healthy despite their low birth weights. If I hadn't delivered when I did, Simon, who had stopped growing at the same rate as the others, may not have made it. The fact that he survived is due to the exemplary care I received from my perinatologist, Dr. Andrew Robertson.

Our babies spent several weeks in the neonatal intensive care unit, mostly to grow, since they had no serious health problems and did not require ventilation to breathe. Today, they are healthy preschoolers with normal development. They are our miracles and the joy of our lives.

I still take a moment each day to remind myself of my infertility journey, and I try not to let the demands of parenting triplets allow me to take them for granted. Despite the fact that I now have the family I always dreamed of, my infertility experience is and always will be part of who I am. Those who have not felt the fear and despair don't understand what it's like not to be able to conceive or carry a baby to term. They don't know how hard it is to accept that your body can't always do what you expect it to do. They haven't experienced the grief that comes from mourning children you may never have. And they don't realize how much discipline it takes to get through the grueling and time-consuming treatments.

Since the birth of my children, I have counseled my sister, two cousins, and several close friends through infertility treatments, and have re-lived my own experience vicariously through them. Although each woman has her own unique story, the infertility experience bonds us together like no other, and we are grateful for this sisterhood.

My Wish for You

It is my hope that this book will comfort you on your journey through infertility. I hope it will help you understand the causes of infertility and how it is treated. I have been where you are now, and I understand how the inability to have the family you desire can become a life crisis. It can affect all aspects of your life—from your career to your relationships with family members and friends. Remember that it is important to get the support you need as you navigate the course of infertility treatment. It also is essential to become empowered with accurate information about the medical options available to you.

—Melanie Morrissey Clark

I know that each and every patient who has difficulty conceiving undergoes both physical and emotional changes that are likely to remain with them for the rest of their lives. In my experience, one of the greatest emotional problems is fear, especially the fear of never being able to conceive.

One of my purposes in writing this book was to share some of my patients' experiences and feelings about their diagnoses and treatment. I tell patients who have not yet started treatment or have to this point been unsuccessful that we are making tremendous strides every day in both the diagnosis of fertility problems and the treatment of disease processes. In the past ten years, we have seen very significant strides in the treatment of male factor infertility. For example, we can now directly inject the sperm into the egg in order to achieve fertilization. This has opened the door to many couples who previously had no hope. We have also seen the development of new medias that allow us to grow the embryos out to the blastocyst stage for use with in vitro fertilization, allowing us to choose more carefully which embryos are most likely to implant. This has helped us significantly decrease the number of embryos we transfer and significantly decrease the multiple gestation rate. The future certainly holds great promise.

—C. Maud Doherty, M.D.

1

Infertility—An Overview

For most couples, one of the most difficult things about having a fertility problem is facing it. Most of us grow up assuming we can have children. We believe childbearing is a sort of birthright, and we are often shocked and traumatized when that birthright is threatened by our inability to conceive. It is estimated that one out of every ten couples of reproductive age—6.1 million people in the United States—experience some form of infertility.

Research shows that the women most likely to have trouble conceiving are those in the 35 to 44 age group. Infertility rates start to increase around age 35 and continue to increase as women reach age 40 and beyond. In fact, only 2 percent of babies are born to women over age 40.

Gender equality is alive and well when it comes to physical causes of infertility. About 40 percent of a couple's infertility problems can be attributed to a female factor and about 40 percent to a male factor. The remaining 20 percent of cases are attributed to a combined male-female factor or to unexplained infertility.

Defining Infertility

Primary Infertility

The term *primary infertility* describes those who have never been able to achieve a pregnancy or carry a pregnancy to term. Medically, infertility is considered a disease. It is defined as the inability to conceive after one year of well-timed, unprotected intercourse or the inability to carry a pregnancy to term. The accepted rule of thumb for when to seek fertility treatment is after a couple fails to achieve a pregnancy after one year of unprotected intercourse. Women who are over age 35 or who have a history of irregular cycles or known infertility risk factors should see a doctor sooner. Men who have hernia repairs, undescended testicles, or an injury to the scrotal area should have a sperm count done before waiting one year.

Secondary Infertility

Past fertility does not guarantee future fertility. Some couples discover their fertility problem when trying to conceive a second time; they realize they may have been fortunate with the conception of their first baby. Today, most physicians define *secondary infertility* as the inability to conceive after previously having carried a pregnancy to term. Some couples experience both primary and secondary infertility. Surprisingly, secondary infertility is as common as primary infertility, accounting for a large percentage of those seeking treatment in fertility clinics across the country.

Societal Influences

A variety of societal influences have contributed to the rise of infertility.

- *The changing roles and aspirations of women.* Today, 53 million women in the United States earn a paycheck. For many, work is invigorating and rewarding enough to put off starting a family.

- *Delayed childbearing* . On average, women have their first child three years later than they did twenty years ago. Studies show fertility declines with age, falling dramatically after age 35.

- *Increased use of contraceptives.* Widespread use of condoms and birth control pills has resulted in fewer accidental pregnancies—allowing individuals to make a conscious decision to start a family when they are financially and psychologically ready; as a result, women are often older and may have trouble conceiving.

- *More sexually transmitted diseases* (*STDs*). Increased rates of STDs which, when left untreated, lead to more infertility.

> *Our infertility experience has made me and my husband closer. He reassures me that he married me because of our love for each other no matter what—kids or no kids.*
>
> *Anne, 30*
> *Diagnosis: endometriosis*

- *Environmental toxins.* More toxins exist in today's environment than ever before, and some are thought to have an effect on fertility and miscarriage.

Seeking Treatment

As a result of factors such as these, more than 1 million couples seek treatment for infertility every year. Of those seeking help today, most need only minimal intervention, such as medications to help women ovulate regularly. But for about 40,000 couples each year, high-tech assisted reproduction is their only hope. More than 50 percent of couples who receive good medical care from an infertility specialist will be successful in achieving a pregnancy and live birth.

2

Female Infertility:
Risk Factors and Causes

When she had trouble getting pregnant, Sandy couldn't help but feel it was somehow her fault. She hadn't been promiscuous before her marriage, but there was always the chance that an old boyfriend had given her a sexually transmitted disease that had gone undiagnosed. Or maybe the occasional cigarette and heavy drinking in college were to blame. Sandy was sure she would never have children, and that she herself had destroyed her fertility. The guilt weighed heavily on Sandy's mind, making it difficult for her to enjoy her once-fulfilling career and quiet dinners with her husband. "If I never have a baby, I will never forgive myself," she said.

Risk Factors for Female Infertility

When faced with the possibility of a fertility problem, many of us often ask, "Why me?" The tendency to place blame is strong, and most point the finger at themselves. But the truth is, infertility is the result of a medical problem. Still, several lifestyle factors can influence fertility.

Smoking and Alcohol/Drugs

Lifestyle choices such as smoking cigarettes and abusing alcohol and drugs can take their toll on fertility.

Smoking, which has long been known to increase the risk of ectopic (tubal) pregnancy, diminishes a woman's fertility by disrupting hormone levels and making embryo implantation difficult. Smokers are, in fact, four times more likely to take longer than a year to conceive than are nonsmokers. In addition, cigarette smoking can cause female infertility by hastening menopause, according to researchers at Massachusetts General Hospital; the researchers established a direct connection between the chemicals in cigarette smoke and the genetic signals that cause ovarian cells to die.

How could this be? You grow up, fall in love and want a family. I felt like less of a woman because I could not conceive. Now that I have twins, I thank God every day.
Joann, 32
Diagnosis: unexplained infertility

Alcohol has also been shown to affect fertility. Findings from a 1998 study published in the *British Medical Journal* reveal that even moderate drinking could cut a woman's chance for conception by as much as 50 percent. The researchers theorize that alcohol interferes with ovulation and egg transportation. Some studies have suggested that high caffeine intake can cause infertility in women as well, so many specialists suggest couples eliminate caffeine from their diets while trying to conceive and during pregnancy.

Exercise and Diet

Women who carry physical fitness to excess may harm their reproductive functions. For example, excessive exercise and rigorous dieting may impair a woman's ability to ovulate if her overall amount of body fat is greatly reduced; a lack of body fat can diminish the supply of the hormone *estrogen*, which is important for ovulation and menstruation. The result may be *anovulation*—no eggs are released from the ovary—and scanty or missed periods. Some research suggests that ovulation problems in exercising women may be due to nutritional problems, as well.

Sexually Transmitted Diseases (STDs)

Sexually transmitted diseases (STDs) are a primary cause of infertility among both women and men today. Each year in the United States, doctors diagnose more than 4 million cases of chlamydia, 1 million cases of gonorrhea, and more than 10 million viral infections.

Left untreated, STDs can cause *pelvic inflammatory disease (PID)*, leading to scar tissue formation and damage to the delicate membranes lining the fallopian tubes. This condition makes it difficult or impossible for an egg to travel through the tubes. With each episode of an STD, the chances of damage to the reproductive system increase.

Perhaps the most damaging STD for women is *chlamydia*, also known as the "silent infection" because three out of four infected women won't have early symptoms. Two out of five infected women will develop PID. Twenty percent of the time, PID leads to infertility. Eighteen percent of women will have chronic pelvic pain, and 9 percent of the time they will have a life-threatening tubal pregnancy. The more sexual partners a woman has had, the greater her risk of being exposed to chlamydia.

Stress and Psychological Factors

In some cases, chronic stress may cause erratic hormone levels in women, which can disrupt ovulation. Acute stress can even result in a woman not ovulating or missing her period. Infertility certainly causes emotional distress, and one study found that the depression women experience while dealing with infertility is the same as that of women dealing with cancer. Learning relaxation techniques such as meditation and yoga may help couples cope with infertility.

Causes of Female Infertility

Age

The "fertility clock" ticks quickly for women, making a woman's age the single most important factor in whether she can conceive and deliver a healthy baby. Women are born with their full complement of eggs—several million—in their ovaries. However, as a woman ages, the number of eggs she carries quickly declines. In fact, by puberty, the average woman has only about 300,000 left. Aging not only affects the number of eggs in the ovaries but also the quality of the eggs and their ability to create healthy embryos. In older women, compromised embryo quality contributes to a higher miscarriage rate.

Despite increased publicity about the link between infertility and age, many professional women are delaying childbirth. Many women are unaware of how early their ability to conceive may be compromised. Generally, a woman is most fertile in her

Decline in Female Egg Supply

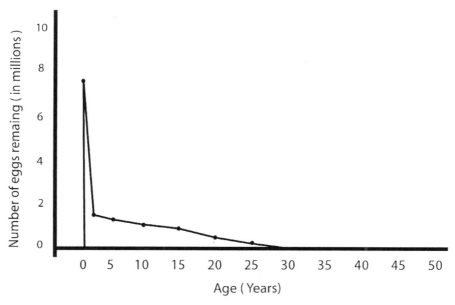

At birth, women are born with their entire supply of eggs. They may have as many as 7 million at birth. This number declines to about 300,000 during puberty and, by her late 30s, a woman has only a few thousand.

20s. Her fertility declines as she reaches her 30s, and particularly after age 35. After age 40, the decline is dramatic. Women in their late 30s are often surprised to learn that even though they are having regular menstrual cycles, their reproductive system may already have been compromised.

Still, there is room for optimism. Women are having their first babies in their 30s and even 40s, usually with donor eggs, thanks to advances in fertility treatments. Blood tests taken at certain times during a woman's cycle can evaluate her ovarian reserve—the quantity and health of eggs left in the ovary. These tests can help a physician determine whether age has become a factor in a woman's infertility.

Endometriosis

Endometriosis affects an estimated 40 to 60 percent of female infertility patients. The disease develops when menstrual blood and tissue, which normally leaves the body during a woman's period, backs up into the fallopian tubes and flows out into the pelvic cavity. *Endometrial cells* then implant on the ovaries and surrounding tissue. Symptoms include:

- severe menstrual cramps
- heavy menstrual bleeding
- lower back pain
- ovulation pain
- painful bowel movements
- pelvic cysts and tumors
- painful intercourse
- difficulty conceiving
- recurring bladder infections

Blood-filled ovarian cysts called *endometriomas* often form, leading to poor-quality egg development and, possibly, inhibiting egg release. Endometriosis may also cause the formation of scar tissue that obstructs the ends of the fallopian tubes and inhibits fertilization. Women with severe endometriosis may have completely or partially blocked tubes, rendering natural conception almost impossible, while women with moderate or minimal endometriosis may have only ovulation or fertilization problems. Patients with endometriosis

Female Reproductive System

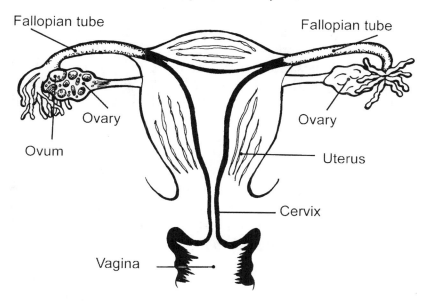

also have elevated levels of *macrophages*, or specialized cells which are thought to inhibit a sperm's ability to penetrate an egg.

Although the cause of endometriosis is not known, it is thought to be a progressive disease, worsening with age. Some evidence suggests that endometriosis runs in families. The only way to diagnose endometriosis is through a *laparoscopy*. This surgical procedure is performed on an outpatient basis. It requires a small incision near the navel so the surgeon can use a viewing scope to visualize the insides of the pelvic cavity and outer walls of the uterus and fallopian tubes. The procedure allows for the biopsy of suspicious lesions.

Many women keep this disease in check by taking birth control pills until they are ready to conceive. Hormones in the pills halt ovulation and produce lighter, sporadic, or even absent periods, decreasing the chance for new lesions to develop; the progesterone component of the pill also causes the atrophy of the glandular implants of endometriosis. The disease can also be controlled and treated with surgery and medical therapy.

Cervical Factor

The cervical factor accounts for about 5 percent of all female infertility problems. The *cervix*, located in the lower part of the uterus, contains a canal through which sperm enter the uterine cavity and ultimately reach the fallopian tube to fertilize an egg. If the *cervical mucus* (which helps transport the sperm) is compromised, the sperm may have difficulty traveling through this canal.

A variety of conditions can affect the cervical mucus. For example, some women have sperm *antibodies* in their cervical mucus. Sperm antibodies result from the body attacking its cells as if they were foreign materials or bacteria. In the case of sperm antibodies in the cervical mucus, antibodies attach to a sperm, killing or immobilizing it. In other cases, ovulation-stimulating drugs are known to thicken cervical mucus, making it difficult for sperm to swim through the canal. More information on this drug side effect is covered in chapter 4.

Another cervical problem, *cervical stenosis*, is a condition in which the opening into the uterus is restricted. This is often caused by scarring and narrowing of the cervical opening, and sperm transport is hampered.

DES Exposure and Previous Surgeries

Exposure to the medication DES (diethylstilbestrol) while in the womb is another risk factor for infertility. This medication was given to pregnant women in the 1950s and 1960s to help prevent miscarriage. Individuals who were exposed to this drug while in their mother's uterus may have abnormalities of their own reproductive tracts. In some women this may mean a small, T-shaped uterus or an abnormal cervical opening.

Another risk factor for women is previous abdominal or pelvic surgery, which may have caused scarring or pelvic adhesions that might affect fertility.

Uterine Factor

Uterine problems can make it difficult for an embryo to implant and continue growing. Some women are born with abnormalities of the uterus that make it difficult to implant and/or carry a baby to term.

A lot more people have fertility problems than you might think. Once you've been through it, you can empathize with others. You have to listen to your heart, not what others say.

Ellene, 35
Diagnosis: failure to ovulate

Benign growths in the uterus, such as polyps and fibroids, also can be problematic. *Polyps,* or small growths, can appear inside the uterus and can contribute to embryo implantation problems. *Fibroids,* or muscle tumors, can develop in the uterine muscle and connective tissue. Depending on their size and location on the uterine wall, fibroids may have to be removed to improve fertility.

If the uterine lining does not become thick enough under hormonal stimulation, the risk of poor implantation and miscarriage may be higher as well.

Hormonal Dysfunction

The proper balance of reproductive hormones in a woman is critical in order for ovulation, conception, and pregnancy to occur. The levels of five major hormones should rise and fall in a distinct pattern throughout a woman's monthly cycle, ultimately causing her to ovulate.

- *FSH (Follicle-Stimulating Hormone).* Secreted by the pituitary gland, FSH stimulates follicle growth. (The follicle is a fluid-filled sac that contains the egg.)
- *LH (Luteinizing Hormone).* Also secreted by the pituitary gland, this hormone causes the follicle to release a mature egg.
- *GnRH (Gonadotropin-Releasing Hormone).* This hormone is responsible for stimulating the release of FSH and LH into the bloodstream.
- *Estrogen.* Secreted by the ovaries, this hormone, along with progesterone, promotes development of a healthy uterine lining.
- *Progesterone.* Produced after ovulation, this hormone prepares the uterine lining for implantation of the embryo and helps maintain the pregnancy.

An imbalance in any of these hormones can cause a woman to ovulate abnormally or not at all. A combination of menstrual history, blood tests, basal body temperature charts, and ultrasound can typically determine whether or not a woman is ovulating.

Thyroid-Related Hormone Problems

Abnormalities in thyroid function or a higher than normal level of the hormone *prolactin*, secreted by the pituitary gland, can also affect fertility. Prolactin is responsible for triggering breast milk production. If elevated, it can disturb ovulation patterns and cause problems in the latter two weeks of the cycle—the luteal phase—and ultimately result in a poor uterine environment for implantation. If a woman has *hyperthyroidism* (too much thyroid hormone) or *hypothyroidism* (too little thyroid hormone), she will need to take medication to correct the imbalance, optimizing fertility and possibly reducing the risk of miscarriage.

Polycystic Ovary Syndrome (PCOS)

The most common hormonal imbalance among women of reproductive age is *polycystic ovary syndrome*, or *PCOS*. A common cause of infertility, the syndrome gets its name from the small cysts that form in the ovaries when a woman's ovulation process is not functioning correctly. Symptoms of this condition can include irregular or absent periods, infertility, excessive body hair, acne, obesity, and insulin resistance. It is estimated that as many as 10 million women suffer from PCOS in the United States alone. The syndrome is diagnosed by a combination of medical history, a physical, lab tests, and ultrasound. Its symptoms can be treated with medication. Like other hormonal dysfunctions, PCOS can usually be treated with exercise and diet, fertility drugs and insulin-altering agents to achieve pregnancy.

Ultrasound of a Cystic Ovary   **Ultrasound of a Normal Ovary**

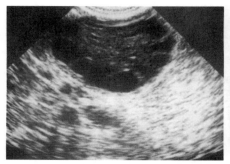   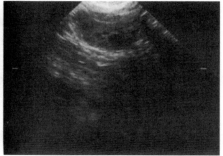

The ovary is the darker mass toward the top of the photo. Note how cysts cluster around the edge of the ovary, giving it a black "pearl necklace" appearance.

The normal ovary has a more consistent appearance, with only scattered follicles, as indicated in the small follicle in the lower right-hand edge of the ovary. *Photos courtesy of Richard Legro, M.D., Pennsylvania State College of Medicine.*

Tubal Scarring and Pelvic Adhesions

Tubal scarring is not uncommon following an episode of pelvic inflammatory disease and can even be caused by an undetected infection after an elective abortion or asymptomatic chlamydia. Women with tubal scarring are at high risk for an ectopic (tubal) pregnancy, where the fertilized egg gets caught in one of the woman's two fallopian tubes on its way to the uterus. An embryo that grows undetected in the tube can result in the loss of that tube, making it more difficult for a woman to achieve a subsequent pregnancy on her own. Tubal pregnancy occurs in about one out of every ninety pregnancies in the United States. If left untreated, this condition can cause severe bleeding into the pelvic cavity, shock, and even death.

Pelvic adhesions—fibrous bands that form between pelvic structures or block the fallopian tubes from picking up the egg—have a variety of causes. These include a ruptured appendix, other previous surgery, endometriosis, and pelvic infection. Unfortunately, most severe pelvic adhesions cannot be successfully treated with further surgery and the surgery itself can result in still more scarring. Usually, if adhesions are severe, a physician will recommend in vitro fertilization to achieve a pregnancy by bypassing the blocked fallopian tubes. In vitro fertilization involves fertilization of the eggs outside the woman's body, followed by transferring fertilized eggs (embryos) to the uterus for implantation.

Premature Ovarian Failure

All ovaries stop functioning eventually, but some women's ovaries fail earlier than expected. *Premature ovarian failure* is defined as the loss of ovarian function before age 40. Some women with this problem will continue to have menstrual cycles and others will have irregular or no cycles. Menopausal symptoms may appear suddenly or they may appear more gradually. Women with premature ovarian failure who produce eggs usually have poor quality eggs and consequently more embryos that do not implant well. If a woman with ovarian failure gets pregnant with her own eggs, her risk of miscarriage may be higher due to the chromosomal changes that often occur in the egg(s).

A woman might have ovarian failure for several reasons. These include previous radiation, chemotherapy for cancer, an inherited disposition to undergo early menopause, or *autoimmune disorders*, caused when the body's immune system destroys normal body tissue. In most cases, ovarian failure is unexplainable. Blood tests to check the levels of the hormones FSH and LH drawn on day 2 or 3 of a woman's cycle can tell a doctor if a woman is experiencing premature ovarian failure. Unfortunately, there is no treatment for this condition. Women who experience ovarian failure may want to consider using donor eggs to achieve a pregnancy.

Multiple Miscarriage

For some women, the problem is not getting pregnant, but rather maintaining the pregnancy. One in six of all pregnancies ends in miscarriage before 12 weeks, and most of these are caused by random abnormalities in the chromosomes in the embryo. Some women experience multiple pregnancy losses. For more details on pregnancy loss, see chapter 10.

Unexplained Infertility

Unexplained infertility is basically a diagnosis of exclusion. Once a physician has thoroughly excluded all other causes for infertility and a couple is still unable to conceive, the diagnosis is unexplained infertility. About 10 percent of couples fall into this category.

Under these circumstances, the couple may be advised to move quickly to assisted reproductive technologies—such as in vitro fertilization—in order to determine whether an egg/sperm interaction, or quality of sperm or egg problem, may exist. Couples with unexplained infertility have a 40 to 60 percent conception rate within four years. Success rates for concrete diagnoses vary, depending on the severity of the disease process present and whether the patients are willing to undergo advanced treatment.

Secondary Infertility

With a few exceptions, secondary infertility can have the same causes as primary infertility. In some cases the condition may have always been present, but the couple was fortunate to have conceived previously. Endometriosis, which may progress over time, is a common cause of secondary infertility in women. Age is often a factor as well; couples starting families later in life who wish to space their children's births by several years may find themselves facing secondary infertility as the mother's age advances beyond 35. In rare cases, the problem may be the result of complications with a previous pregnancy, changes in general health, or use of medications.

3

Getting a Diagnosis

Susan was nervous about her first appointment with her reproductive endocrinologist, but was pleasantly surprised to find the initial appointment was easy. She filled out a fertility evaluation form, answered questions about her health and menstrual history, and underwent a standard physical examination. "When I left the office, I was surprised at how hopeful I felt. Just talking with a professional and taking that first step felt like a weight had been lifted off my shoulders. Now, at least, I was taking action, and I felt ready to begin the process of diagnosing and treating whatever was keeping me from becoming pregnant."

The Fertility Evaluation

Obtaining an infertility diagnosis begins with a series of tests. Because at least 20 percent of all fertility problems can be attributed to *both* the man and the woman, it's important for both partners to get a fertility evaluation as soon as possible. More information on evaluation of the male partner appears in chapter eight.

Most physicians first ask couples to fill out a *fertility evaluation form*. In order to obtain a detailed medical history and lifestyle assessment, questions are asked of both the man and woman. Included are questions pertaining to:

- Age.
- Caffeine, alcohol and drug use, including prescription drugs. Caffeine may be associated with an increased risk of miscarriage. Barbiturates can decrease or inhibit the hormone GnRH, which regulates other hormones related to egg production.
- Exposure to chemicals, toxins, or radiation in the work environment.
- Smoking history.
- Marital history. Number of years, types of contraception used.
- Sexual intercourse. Frequency, difficulties, coital positions, adequate penetration, ejaculation, pain or discomfort, and type of lubrication used.
- History of any significant health problems or surgeries.
- Types of birth control used in the past.
- History of sexually transmitted diseases.
- Pregnancy history. Dates, outcomes, miscarriages, abortions, complications, number of naturally conceived children.
- Previous marriages. Contraception, children, miscarriages.
- Menstrual history (age at onset, length, duration, vaginal discharge).
- Past infertility tests (dates, results).
- Past infertility treatments.
- Basic medical history. Allergies, medications.

A thorough physical exam for the woman should follow the written evaluation. This exam should include a cervical screening for chlamydia and gonorrhea, if appropriate, as well as for other potentially harmful genital organisms. The bacterial screening may include testing for *ureaplasma* and *mycoplasma*, organisms that may cause early miscarriage. Some clinics or doctors will test for these organisms by taking vaginal cultures or cultures from the penis.

Blood samples may be tested for hepatitis B and C, HIV, rubella, blood type/Rh, and any other indicated concerns. A test for levels of FSH and *estradiol* on the second or third day of a woman's cycle can help the doctor estimate the ovarian reserve.

A complete medical history and physical, as well as a complete menstrual history, will usually determine whether or not a woman is ovulating. The woman may be asked to do temperature charts or use ovulation predictor kits to help delineate the ovulation pattern.

At-Home Tests

Basal Body Temperature

Some women may be asked to record their *basal body temperature (BBT)*, the body's temperature at rest. This requires taking one's temperature every day before getting out of bed and charting the results for an entire menstrual cycle, beginning on day one (the first day of her period). Drops in body temperature may occur just before ovulation, while a distinct rise should appear just after the egg is released. Experts suggest a couple try to conceive around the time a woman's temperature drops and rises. In most women, this occurs between day 12 and 15 of the cycle. It usually takes two to three months to get an accurate picture of when a woman typically ovulates within her cycle.

Ovulation Predictor Kits (OPKs)

Called *OPKs, ovulation predictor kits* also chart a woman's ovulatory pattern. OPK tests are used on a woman's early-morning urine to measure her LH level and are considered more accurate than the BBT. Since LH is the hormone released just before ovulation, these tests help pinpoint a woman's most fertile time. Although more expensive than using a BBT chart, OPKs are sold over the counter and are easy to use.

The kits instruct you to urinate on the test stick, and about 2 minutes later, it will show whether you are having an LH surge by measuring the amount of LH in your urine. Usually, there are two lines on the test stick—the test line and the control line. If the test line is a lighter shade than the control line, you are not having an LH surge. If the test line is the same or a shade darker than the control line, an LH surge has been detected. Once the LH surge has been detected, you will most likely ovulate within the next 24 hours.

Ask your doctor questions from the start. I trusted my first doctor for too long before I went to another one. So much valuable time was wasted. Ask people in the medical field who they would recommend.

Barb, 36,
mother of a 5-year-old
and pregnant
Diagnosis: secondary
infertility

To ensure you catch the LH surge, you should begin testing a few days before you think you are going to ovulate. If you are taking fertility medication, talk to your doctor about when you should start testing, since fertility medication can change the length of your cycle or affect the test by causing a false positive. Women on fertility drugs or those women with polycystic ovary syndrome may experience an LH surge despite the absence of a mature follicle egg.

Saliva Ovulation Test

A relatively new at-home test, the saliva-based ovulation test, is another option for determining whether ovulation is occurring. Scientists have long known that as estrogen surges the salt content of saliva increases. When the saliva dries, salt crystals are visible under a microscope; they leave a pattern called ferning (the pattern resembles a fern plant).

The saliva ovulation tester is a round device that pairs tiny slides with a handheld microscope. You touch a little brush to saliva in your mouth, then dab it onto a slide. When the saliva is dry, you examine the slide with the microscope. If the salt crystals appear only as small dots, you are not near ovulation. However, if the salt crystals form a chain, or a fern pattern, then ovulation is imminent.

Researchers say the saliva-based test may give you advance warning that you are about to ovulate as you watch the pattern gradually appear. The test is thought to be about 90 percent accurate.

Diagnostic Tests

Hysterosalpingography (HSG)

One of the first tests in an infertility evaluation is a *hysterosalpingography (HSG)*, which studies the woman's upper reproductive tract by x-raying the uterus and fallopian tubes.

The HSG helps diagnose tubal blockage and uterine defects such as polyps, scar tissue, fibroid tumors, or abnormally shaped uterine cavities.

For this test, a *radiopaque dye* is injected through the cervical canal, into the uterus and fallopian tubes. This special dye appears white on the X-ray. The dye reveals the shape of the inside of the uterus and whether the fallopian tubes are open. The optimum time to perform an HSG is just after a patient has finished menstruating and before ovulation.

In addition to being used to diagnose infertility problems, HSGs are ordered for patients with abnormal uterine bleeding and repetitive pregnancy loss.

In some cases, the test can be therapeutic as well as diagnostic. Researchers at the University of Texas Southwestern Medical Center in Dallas studied 132 women with a history of infertility who had HSGs and found that almost 30 percent conceived within three months of having the test. The researchers concluded that the dye may exert enough pressure to clear tiny, often undetectable blockages in the fallopian tubes.

> *I wished the doctors could have found something wrong with me. Each month when my pregnancy test was negative or my menses occurred, it was an emotional upheaval. I kept thinking, "If only...."*
>
> *Rose, 32*
> *Diagnosis: unexplained fertility*

Although an HSG can rule out blocked tubes, it's important to remember that open tubes may not be functional tubes. In some cases further tests may be necessary.

Many physicians recommend patients take ibuprofen before an HSG and have someone accompany them to the procedure because they may experience lower abdominal cramping afterward. Antibiotics may be given for one to three days after the HSG to prevent infection.

Transvaginal Ultrasound

A *pelvic* or *transvaginal ultrasound* is an important part of a woman's evaluation. In fact, most fertility specialists will perform this test during a woman's first visit. High-frequency sound waves produce clear, sharp pictures of the woman's pelvic organs and can reveal any small, benign tumors embedded in the uterine lining. The ultrasound also makes it possible for the physician to examine the thickness of the uterine lining, and any uterine abnormalities or ovarian cysts. Development of the follicle also can be followed with transvaginal ultrasound. To easily determine whether follicles of the correct size are being produced, a physician will perform the ultrasound 15 days before a woman's expected menses, which should be just prior to ovulation. The follicle, a fluid-filled sac containing the egg, should be 18 to 25 millimeters at the time of ovulation.

Sonohysterosalpingogram

A *sonohysterosalpingogram* (SSG), or saline sonogram/ultrasound, detects tiny polyps, fibroids, or scar tissue in the uterine cavity. During the procedure, a tiny catheter is placed into the vagina and then into the uterus. A sterile saline (salt water) solution is then allowed to flow into the uterus while ultrasound is being done. The saline solution expands the uterine cavity, making it easier for the physician to see any defects inside the cavity or on the inner uterine walls. This test complements the HSG since it provides more detailed information about the endometrial cavity.

Hormone Screenings

Hormones are studied through blood tests. A woman's hormones affect every phase of her menstrual cycle, playing a key role in fertility. If the hormone levels are not rising and falling correctly, ovulation and the ability to conceive can be diminished or even eliminated. Actual ovulation occurs 34 to 36 hours after the onset of the luteinizing hormone (LH) surge.

Screening a woman's hormone levels during the first three phases tells a physician whether a woman's cycle is functioning normally. The menstrual cycle consists of four distinct phases:

- The *follicular phase*, during which the follicle develops. This phase is characterized by rising estradiol, which should peak at the time of ovulation. Progesterone levels in the follicular phase are always low. The level of follicular-stimulating hormone (FSH) on day 3 of the cycle is a good predictor of ovarian reserve. Low levels are good; levels between 10 to 15 mlU/ml are considered borderline. Depending on the type of test used and the lab where the test is run, levels between 15 and 25 mlU/ml are problematic. A level above normal indicates the patient has poor ovarian reserve, meaning that her ovaries may not produce good quality eggs.

- *Ovulation*, the time at which the signal to ovulate occurs, as well as actual ovulation. When the LH level rises two to four times above the baseline level, it is considered an ovulatory surge.

- The *luteal phase* begins after ovulation. This phase is characterized by rising progesterone levels and also by a secondary peak of the estradiol level 7 days after ovulation. Progesterone levels are commonly measured 6 to 7 days after ovulation. The basal body temperature will rise .3 to .5 degrees Fahrenheit during this phase. If a pregnancy occurs, the hormone levels and temperature should remain elevated. If no pregnancy occurs, the hormone levels usually drop and menstruation begins.

- The *menstrual phase*, when a drop in hormone levels leads to the onset of menses.

An easy way to estimate the day of ovulation in most women is to subtract 14 days from the total cycle length. Thus, testing hormone levels at certain times during a woman's cycle can determine hormonal function. When necessary, fertility drugs that stimulate production of certain hormones, such as estradiol—the most active estrogen—can help a woman ovulate or maintain an early pregnancy.

Other hormone levels, including those for thyroid-stimulating hormone (TSH) and prolactin, should be checked during an infertility evaluation. If the thyroid produces too much thyroid hormone, *hyperthyroidism* occurs. If the thyroid produces too little, *hypothyroidism* results. Either of these conditions can affect ovulation, and, in the case of hypothyroidism, the miscarriage rate may be increased if the condition is left untreated. Prolactin, a hormone produced by the pituitary gland, is responsible for the induction and maintenance of lactation or breastfeeding. Occasionally, prolactin production will increase in a non-nursing woman. Higher levels can disrupt ovulation patterns. An oral medication is available to correct prolactin levels.

Cervical Mucus and Postcoital Testing

Cervical mucus helps carry swimming sperm through the cervix and into the uterine cavity, where they enter the fallopian tubes to fertilize an egg. Cervical mucus is estrogen dependent, so there should be an increase in mucus production at the time of ovulation.

Some physicians may choose to test a woman's cervical mucus after sexual intercourse to determine whether sperm are swimming freely. Performed on the day the mucus is expected to be most fertile—the day of the LH surge—this test is called the *postcoital test (PCT)*. (This test is no longer used as frequently as it once was. However, some doctors may order it for selected patients.) To complete the test, the couple has intercourse without using vaginal lubrication at the time when the woman is ovulating. A sample of her cervical mucus is taken shortly afterward and examined to see if her partner's sperm can survive in and swim through it. In postcoital testing, a woman's mucus is evaluated for:

- *Consistency*: should be thin and clear.
- *Stretchability*: should stretch an inch without breaking. (This characteristic is called *spinnbarkeit.*)
- *Volume*: should be abundant.
- *pH level*: should be 6.5 to 8.0 (*pH level* refers to whether the mucus is alkaline or acidic. An alkaline environment is better for sperm survival.)
- *Ferning*: a pattern (looks like a fern plant) seen in cervical mucus under a microscope; ferning indicates good estrogen levels and "fertile" mucus.

A postcoital test should be done 6 to 10 hours after intercourse, and the specimen should contain ten or more sperm per

HPF (high-powered microscope field). Ten or more sperm with progressive *motility*, or movement, should be considered an adequate PCT. Proper timing in the woman's cycle is critical for this test to be accurate.

A woman can check her own mucus on day 13 or 14 of her cycle by holding the mucus between the thumb and the forefinger and seeing if the mucus pulls apart like a raw egg white. Mucus that is thin, slippery, stretchy and clear, indicates that a woman is about ready to ovulate and that her cervical mucus is ready to transport sperm to the fallopian tubes.

Endometrial Biopsy

An *endometrial biopsy* helps determine whether the thickness and structure of the endometrium—lining of the uterus—is conducive to implantation. (This is another test that is no longer routinely used to diagnose infertility; however, it may be indicated for patients with regular cycles and recurrent pregnancy loss.) During the procedure, a physician removes a small tissue sample from the endometrium with a narrow catheter that is inserted through the cervix and into the uterus. The sample is sent to a lab for analysis.

This biopsy is also used to diagnose a *luteal phase defect (LPD)*, which would mean that either an inadequate amount of progesterone is being secreted by the *corpus luteum* (the follicle the released egg leaves behind) or that the endometrium is failing to respond to adequate progesterone levels. Progesterone is important in helping the fertilized egg implant in the uterus.

Diagnosis of LPD is made by an endometrial biopsy performed 7 to 12 days after the LH surge. The procedure is done in the doctor's office and is somewhat uncomfortable, so taking ibuprofen 30 minutes before the test is recommended.

An endometrial biopsy may also be done in women with repeated embryo implantation failures to test for the presence of Beta-3 integrin, a cell surface receptor, in the uterine lining. This receptor is thought to be important in the process of implantation.

Laparoscopy and Hysteroscopy

A *laparoscopy* is performed to look for endometriosis, adhesions, fibroids, and abnormalities of the uterus, tubes, or ovaries. It is usually the last step in the fertility evaluation, unless endometriosis or other abnormalities are strongly suspected, in which case it should be done earlier in the diagnostic work up. To begin the procedure, carbon dioxide gas is used to expand the abdominal cavity for better viewing. Then, the physician inserts a long, thin tube called a *laparoscope* into the pelvic cavity through a small incision in the navel. If endometriosis or adhesions are discovered, the surgeon can remove them during the procedure. This surgery is usually done in the follicular or luteal phase of the cycle.

> *I had two children from my previous marriage, but was depressed because my new husband and I wanted a child. It was hard to accept that I was having fertility problems. We were one cycle away from in vitro when I got pregnant.*
>
> *Debbie, 37*
> *eight months pregnant*
> *Diagnosis: secondary infertility.*

Perhaps the most important advantage of laparoscopy is that it eliminates the need for a large pelvic incision. Performed under general anesthesia in a hospital or surgery center on an outpatient basis, this test usually takes under an hour to complete.

Once a woman is alert, able to drink fluids, and urinate, she can go home. The anesthesia may cause grogginess, and abdominal muscles may be sore, so recovery may take several days. The tiny incision will not have a large dressing, so showers are allowed the day following the procedure.

Hysteroscopy is performed to confirm and treat any uterine abnormalities found during an HSG or saline sonogram. During a hysteroscopy, a tiny, telescope-like instrument is inserted through the cervical canal and into the uterus. It gives the doctor a full view of the uterine cavity, allowing him or her to remove any uterine polyps, fibroid tumors, or adhesions. This simple procedure can be performed either using local anesthesia in the doctor's office or general anesthesia. Removal of fibroid tumors requires general anesthesia.

After Diagnostic Testing

Keep in mind that not every woman undergoes each diagnostic test described in this chapter. Your physician will guide you through the tests appropriate for you. Then, once the tests have helped the physician reach a diagnosis, a woman may consider a course of treatment to help her conceive. The options include combinations of medications, surgery, and the newer advanced reproductive technologies, all of which are covered in the chapters ahead.

4

Treatments for Female Infertility

W hen she first started treatment, Christine was uncomfortable with taking drugs to stimulate ovulation and to regulate her erratic hormone levels. The oral drugs didn't bother her much, but when she moved on to injectables, she felt irritable and moody. "My doctor said there is no evidence that these drugs affect disposition, but I found myself crying a lot more than usual. I finally realized that it was mostly because I was upset and worried all the time about whether I'd get pregnant."

Finally, after two rounds of oral drugs and three rounds of injectables, Christine became pregnant and delivered a baby boy. "Without the drugs, I probably would never have become pregnant and maintained my pregnancy through the first trimester. It was all worth it, and I'm already thinking about doing it again for baby number two."

When to Seek a Specialist

Some women should see a fertility specialist sooner than others. A woman who has had irregular cycles or is over age 35 should see a specialist after six months of unprotected intercourse that does not result in pregnancy. Similarly, a woman who has had two or three miscarriages also should see a specialist early.

Any of the following are reasons to visit an infertility specialist:

- The woman is over age 35.
- The woman has a history of pelvic infection, has endometriosis, or has tubal damage from infections or a prior ectopic pregnancy.
- The woman has had three or more miscarriages.
- The woman has an irregular menstrual cycle, and possibly oligo (irregular) ovulation or anovulation (does not ovulate) in response to the fertility drug clomiphene citrate.
- The male partner's semen analysis shows a low sperm count, low motility (motion), poor morphology (shape), or sperm antibodies.
- Results of basic tests for both partners have come back normal despite two years of trying to conceive.

Start Treatment with a Plan

This chapter and the one that follows explore a variety of infertility treatments. Fortunately, many of these treatments often prove successful; however, not every couple succeeds right away. And some may not succeed at all. Whether or not treatments work for a couple, they are costly, both financially and emotionally. For this reason, many experts advise couples to formulate an infertility treatment plan at the start.

Formulating a plan should not cast a cloud of gloom over your hopes. Rather, once a plan is in place, you can rest easy knowing you are prepared to make responsible decisions about your health and finances.

Which Treatments to Undergo

Which treatments are you willing to undergo and for how long? Some couples want to try oral medications but not injectable ones. Others are open to artificial insemination but not in vitro fertilization. Still others are willing to try all treatments with the exception of using donor eggs or sperm. By understanding the various treatment options, you will be in a better position to choose which treatments are appropriate for you. And, talk to your doctor about how long you should continue a line of treatment. For example, how long is it safe to take fertility drugs? Some individuals may jeopardize their health by taking drugs longer than is recommended.

> *The worst part about treatment is finding out you're not pregnant and grieving before you can go on to the next month. There are always tears to be shed for what could have been a new life. It's an emotional struggle.*
>
> *Deb, 34*
> *Diagnosis: unexplained infertility*

Financial Planning

Setting a financial limit is wise. By almost anyone's standards, infertility treatment is expensive. Countless couples have gone into debt in order to try "just one more time." Experts advise against this, saying those who reach this point may be suffering from a compulsion much like any other activity they feel "driven" to accomplish. The compulsion to continue treatment sets in innocently enough. Many infertility patients start out thinking that all they need is a couple of good cycles, a little boost with fertility drugs, and they will take home a baby. Then the monthly cycles can turn into years of "just one more time and we will get pregnant." Accordingly, it helps to have a plan in place, one based on logic rather than unsettled emotions.

Preparing Emotionally

Indeed, making the decision to seek treatment for infertility may bring initial relief and a new sense of hope for becoming a parent. Still, keep in mind that treatment, which may continue for months or years, can be emotionally draining at times. Many patients report going through cycles of optimism and despair as they try another treatment, but are disappointed when conception does not occur.

Seeking a diagnosis and treatment of infertility requires an enormous commitment of time, energy, and resources. Along the way, it is common for patients—both male and female—to experience intense feelings such as irritability, anger, sadness, mild depression, frustration, guilt, and grief. These uncomfortable emotions stem from the persistent and deep-rooted fear that they will never have a child.

Further, moral and spiritual issues can influence decisions about infertility treatment. Some individuals have ethical problems with treatment, particularly with assisted reproductive technologies (ARTs) such as in vitro fertilization. Others may feel that treatment conflicts with their religious beliefs and that if they are meant to have children it will happen without modern technology.

It is best if marital partners are in agreement about treatment. Again, these limits can be agreed upon in advance. The health of the woman or man undergoing treatment should always be a top priority.

Finding the Right Doctor

Because many couples are initially reluctant to acknowledge a possible fertility problem, most begin treatment with the woman's obstetrician-gynecologist, or OB/GYN. An obstetrician is a physician who specializes in the management of pregnancy and childbirth; a gynecologist is a physician specializing in diagnosing and treating problems with the female reproductive system. As long as the OB/GYN proceeds through the basic infertility tests in a timely fashion, there is no need to rush to a specialist. These initial tests typically consist of a hysterosalpingography for the female and a semen analysis for the male. If the physician is reluctant to initiate testing and the couple is concerned about their fertility, a second opinion is in order. Depending on the outcome of the initial tests, the OB/GYN will often refer the couple to an infertility specialist, a *reproductive endocrinologist (RE)*. An RE is an OB/GYN who has completed a fellowship in the sub-specialty of infertility and the hormones of reproduction.

Going through the laparoscopy, the drugs and the emotional trials was worth it. As I sit and look at my little boy, I realize I would do it again if I had to.
Jane, 29
Diagnosis: endometriosis

Credentials of the RE are important. Ask if your RE is *board-certified*. To become a board-certified reproductive endocrinologist (RE), a physician must first have completed requirements to be certified in gynecology and obstetrics; then he or she must complete two or three additional years of fellowship training in the field of infertility or reproductive endocrinology. The physician must then pass a written and oral exam.

Approximately 600 board-certified reproductive endocrinologists practice in the United States. To find a specialist near you, ask for a referral from friends, relatives, or from your primary care physician. You may also wish to check your library for the *American Board of Medical Specialties Directory,* published by Marquis Who's Who or check the Internet at www.abms.org. You may also write for a physician referral list from RESOLVE (www.resolve.org), the infertility patient advocacy group; or visit the Society of Reproductive Endocrinologists Web site at www.asrm.org. More information on these organizations is listed in the Resource section at the back of this book.

Infertility Treatments for Women

Hormonal Drug Therapy

The most common infertility treatment involves hormone regulation through fertility drugs. For many couples, infertility is the result of a hormonal dysfunction that can be corrected with hormonal treatments. The good news is, up to 75 percent of these couples eventually achieve pregnancies. Hormonal treatments typically begin with drug therapy.

Fertility drugs are designed to stimulate ovulation in women and ideally should be prescribed only after completion of a thorough physical evaluation and a hysterosalpingogram (HSG). A cycle of hormone-regulating drugs will do nothing to help a woman whose tubes are completely blocked or whose partner has a very low sperm count. Often, these drugs work hand in hand with other treatments. For example, a woman with severe endometriosis may have surgery to remove scar tissue and endometriosis lesions and then take a cycle of fertility drugs to help achieve a pregnancy. Women who undergo in vitro fertilization also take fertility drugs.

Ovulation-Stimulating Drugs

Clomiphene Citrate

The drug most commonly prescribed for a woman who has ovulatory dysfunction is *clomiphene citrate,* sold under the trade names *Clomid* and *Serophene.* An anti-estrogenic drug, clomiphene citrate blocks the effects of estrogen throughout the body. As a result, the hypothalamus in the brain responds to the low levels of estrogen by releasing more of the hormone GnRH in a pulse-like fashion. GnRH then stimulates the pituitary gland to release LH and FSH, which in turn stimulates the ovary to produce estrogen and eggs.

> *We were about to end treatment. Then, I took Pergonal and got pregnant on the first try. It was our fourth insemination. I'm glad it worked because we could not afford in vitro.*
>
> *Sandy*
> *Diagnosis: anovulatory*

Young women who don't ovulate or who ovulate irregularly due to abnormal LH and FSH secretion are good candidates for clomiphene citrate. The drug can also be effective for women with luteal phase defect (LPD). These women have low levels of progesterone in the luteal phase of the menstrual cycle or have a poor response to the levels of progesterone produced by the ovaries; progesterone helps prepare the endometrium for the implantation of the embryo.

The usual dosage of clomiphene is 50 to 150 milligrams once a day, starting on day 3 or 5 of the cycle and continuing for five days. LH urine kits can be used to monitor ovulation. Some doctors will order an ultrasound to make sure the follicles are developing. Some women may require additional medications to help them ovulate, or release, the eggs.

Women who have no fertility problems other than the lack of or irregular ovulation have an 80 percent chance of ovulating with Clomid and a 50 percent chance of becoming pregnant within six months. Eight to 10 percent of women on Clomid will have a multiple-gestation pregnancy—most likely twins. By comparison, about 1 percent of the general population delivers twins.

Side Effects of Clomiphene

A side effect associated with the use of clomiphene is the drug's effect on the cervical mucus. The mucus may become dry or "hostile" and inhibit the ability of sperm to swim, diminishing chances for fertilization. If this occurs on low doses of clomiphene, increasing the dose will usually make the problem worse.

To overcome this side effect, some physicians use clomiphene in conjunction with artificial insemination if the cervical mucus does not transport sperm. Some physicians will order a postcoital test to check the cervical mucus after intercourse to determine whether or not artificial insemination is necessary.

Clomiphene can also cause significant mood swings in some women. Others report hot flashes, headaches, and breast tenderness.

Injectable Gonadotropins

Not all women respond to the first-line drug therapy, clomiphene citrate. So, other drugs, injectable gonadotropins—also known as "super ovulation" drugs—are commonly prescribed. These drugs do the work of the important sex hormones FSH and LH which would normally be produced by the pituitary gland to stimulate the follicles developing in the ovary. There are two types of injectable gonadotropins—one which contains both LH and FSH and the other which contains mostly FSH.

In the past, injectable gonadotropins were made from the purified urine of menopausal women, who naturally have high levels of FSH and LH because their ovaries are becoming inactive. Nowadays however, these hormones can be genetically engineered, making the drugs more pure. The injectable gonadotropins include *human menopausal gonadotropin (hMG), follicle stimulating hormone (FSH), human chorionic gonadotropin (hCG),* and *gonadotropin releasing hormone (GnRH).*

Some of the older injectable gonadotropins are given IM—*intramuscularly,* usually deep in the muscle of the buttocks with a 1½ inch needle. Most injections today, however, are given SC—*subcutaneously,* just under the skin, using a smaller, ¼ inch needle. Why the two forms of injection? The older gonadotropin shots are given deep in a muscle to avoid an inflammatory or allergic responses that would occur if they were given just under the skin. But since the newer gonado-tropins are more pure, they may be given by subcutaneous injection. The subcutaneous shots, given with small needles, are less painful and less stressful than intramuscular injections. Many women give themselves subcutaneous injections, using the upper thigh or abdominal area as injection sites.

Studies show that absorption is the same in both the older medications and the newer ones. Some obese women, however, may still require injections IM for the best absorption.

Human Menopausal Gonadotropins (hMG)

Human menopausal gonadotropin (hMG) is used to obtain varying degrees of ovarian stimulation. It contains both the hormones FSH and LH. hMG is given daily for seven to twelve days. Brand names include *Pergonal, Humegon,* and *Repronex.* Only Repronex is approved for subcutaneous injection; Pergonal and Humegon are administered intramuscularly. (Humegon is no longer available in the United States.)

FSH

Follicle stimulating hormone (FSH) is often prescribed when a women is not responding to clomiphene therapy. These injections contain FSH and very little LH. It often helps women who have elevated LH levels and lower FSH levels. It is usually administered daily for about a week. Some doctors combine FSH and hMG for optimal egg development. Brand names for FSH include *Follistim, Fertinex, and Gonal-F,* all of which can be given subcutaneously.

Human Chorionic Gonadotropin (hCG)

The hormone *human chorionic gonadotropin (hCG),* is usually not used alone as a fertility drug. When an ovulation-stimulating drug is prescribed, a physician may also order a "trigger" shot of *hCG*, which tells your body to release the egg or eggs that have matured. The trade names for this hormone are *Novarel, Pregnyl,* and *Ovidrel.* hCG is usually taken by intramuscular injection, although Ovidrel has been approved for subcutaneous injection.

Gonadotropin–Releasing Hormone (GnRH)

Rarely used, *gonadotropin-releasing hormone (GnRH)* stimulates the release of FSH and LH. Sold under the brand names *Factrel* and *Lutrepulse,* the medication is given by injection, either IM or SC. In some cases, the medication is delivered through a light-weight intravenous pump, carried on a belt. These drugs are no longer readily available in the United States and are comparatively quite expensive.

Risks of Injectable Gonadotropins

Careful monitoring is important to ensure that gonadotropins are working but not overstimulating the ovaries. Frequent vaginal ultrasounds and blood tests to monitor levels of estrogen are essential tools for assessing how well the stimulating drugs are working. About 90 percent of women ovulate with injectable gonadotropins, and between 20 and 60 percent conceive, depending on such factors as diagnosis, male factor, and age.

Because of concerns about multiple gestations, some doctors will cancel a cycle if a woman's ultrasound shows too many follicles developing. Or, a concerned doctor might decide to "coast" the stimulation—stop administration of the stimulating drugs until the estrogen levels stop increasing, and then resume the drugs. In some cases physicians combine the use of clomiphene citrate and injectable gonadotropins in an effort to limit costs and higher-order multiple gestations—triplets, quadruplets, quintuplets or higher—and simultaneously improve a woman's mucus and endometrial lining.

The risk of multiple births—about 25 percent—is a side effect of using these drugs. Physicians have the option to cancel the cycle or convert it to an *in vitro fertilization (IVF) cycle* if there are too many mature follicles. Because an IVF cycle involves removing eggs from the woman's body before fertilizing them, it allows a doctor more control over how many embryos are inserted into the uterus, reducing the risk of multiple conceptions. The doctor also has the option of aspirating, or removing, the mature eggs to reduce the number available for fertilization.

Side Effects of Injectable Gonadotropins

Several side effects are possible with injectable gonadotropins. A woman may experience soreness at the site of injection, bloating, and abdominal tenderness. Injectable gonadotropins may heighten emotions in some women. The stress of daily injections, along with financial and psychological pressures, may play a role in mood swings.

A rare but possible side effect of these drugs is *ovarian hyperstimulation*. This occurs in about 1 to 5 percent of stimulated cycles, particularly in women with polycystic ovary syndrome (PCOS). The ovaries enlarge and produce more follicles, resulting in a buildup of fluid in the abdominal cavity. Symptoms usually occur about 7 to 9 days after the trigger shot of hCG or ovulation. In mild cases there may be some abdominal bloating and discomfort. In severe cases there may be large amounts of fluid in the abdomen that can cause breathing difficulties, more than a pound a day in weight gain and, in some cases, a drop in urine output. Severe cases require hospitalization to correct fluid and electrolyte imbalances.

Cost and Availability of Injectable Gonadotropins

The injectable drugs Pergonal, Repronex, Follistim, Fertinex, and Gonal-F are available in the United States. Some U.S. patients legally obtain them from England, Mexico, or Israel because they are less expensive. Although people purchase the drugs outside the United States, patients are treated and monitored in this country by their own physicians. The Food and Drug Administration (FDA) allows patients with prescriptions to bring a two-month supply into the United States for personal use.

Drugs purchased in the United States can cost as much as $2,000 to $3,000 per cycle, depending on the prescribed dosage. Each physician will have his or her own opinion of which medication is best for each patient. An injectable gonadotropin cycle does not just include the drugs, however. Office visits, lab tests, and ultrasounds can add another $1,000 to $1,500 in costs per cycle. Insurance coverage of these medications varies widely.

Other Fertility Drugs

GnRH Agonists

If a woman who is undergoing ovulation induction with injectable gonadotropins has a premature spontaneous midcycle hormonal surge, most of the eggs will fail to mature. To prevent this, *gonadotropin-releasing hormone (GnRH) agonists* may be given. Agonists inhibit ovulation by blocking the brain's ability to stimulate the release of LH and FSH. Agonists cause an initial surge, or "flare," in LH, but then signal the pituitary gland to "turn off" the surge. The drug stops a woman's normal ovulatory cycle so it can be replaced by the artificial one, ensuring a physician greater clinical control of the cycle. A family of synthetic hormones, GnRH agonists may be given for several weeks or for a few days prior to starting the ovulatory stimulating drugs. Commonly used agonists are *leuprolide acetate (Lupron)* and *nafarelin acetate (Synarel)*. Lupron is given by subcutaneous injection. Synarel is administered as a nasal spray.

> *It was difficult watching my wife go through all the treatments. I hated giving her shots and waiting for test results. It made me anxious, and I felt so helpless.*
> *Fred, 37*
> *father of triplets*

Lupron is also prescribed for women with endometriosis or fibroids. The drug can temporarily alleviate a condition that may be preventing pregnancy. The drug inhibits estrogen production, which helps shrink the size of endometriosis lesions on or near the reproductive organs, or to shrink fibroid tumors in the uterus. Estrogen stimulates the growth of endometriosis and fibroids.

GnRH Antagonists

GnRH antagonists are also designed to suppress the FSH and LH surge. Newer than the agonists, the antagonists suppress the surge immediately rather than gradually. *Ganirelix acetate* is sold under the brand name *Antagon*; another drug, *cetrorelix acetate*, is marketed as *Cetrotide*. Both these drugs are taken by injection after the ovulatory stimulating drugs are initiated.

Both GnRH agonists and antagonists can have side effects. If used for longer periods of time, these drugs can cause "medical menopause," producing such symptoms as hot flashes and vaginal dryness.

Progesterone

Progesterone is a hormone produced naturally by the ovaries. Because some women produce inadequate amounts of this hormone, progesterone supplements can be given to enhance the chances of a fertilized egg implanting and surviving.

Used in the luteal phase (after ovulation), progesterone supplements support the endometrial lining, thereby helping an embryo successfully implant and/or supporting an implanted embryo to maintain a pregnancy. Progesterone supplements are particularly effective for women with luteal phase defects who may become pregnant but miscarry so early they are not even aware of the pregnancy.

Progesterone (*Prometrium*) supplements may be taken orally in tablet form, by vaginal suppository or by an IM injection. Progesterone is given either once or twice a day and can be continued into the first trimester of pregnancy, depending on a particular fertility clinic's protocol.

Cancer Risks from Fertility Drugs

No conclusive research to date shows that fertility drugs cause cancer; however, the FDA requires many fertility drugs to carry a warning that they may increase the risk of ovarian cancer. Due to these concerns, many physicians limit use of the drugs. Current recommendations are three to four ovulatory cycles of Clomid.

Commonly Prescribed Drugs for Infertility

Trade Name	Generic Name	Drug Form
Clomid®	clomiphene citrate	tablet
Serophene®	clomiphene citrate	tablet
Follistim™	genetically engineered FSH	subcutaneous injection
Gonal-F®	genetically engineered FSH	subcutaneous injection
Fertinex™	purified FSH from women's urine	subcutaneous injection
Ovidrel	hCG	subcutaneous injection
Pregnyl®	hCG	intramuscular injection
Noravel	hCG	intramuscular injection
Pergonal®	hMG-menotropins	intramuscular injection
Humegon™	hMG-menotropins	intramuscular injection
Lupron®	Leuprolide Acetate-GnRH analogue	subcutaneous injection
Lupron Depot®	Leuprolide Acetate-GnRH analogue	intramuscular injection
Repronex	Menotropins	subcutaneous injection or intramuscular injection
Synarel®	Nafarelin Acetate-GnRH analogue	nasal spray
Zoladex®	Gosereline Acetate-GnRH analogue	subcutaneous injection
Parlodel®	bromocriptine	capsules or tablets
Factrel	GnRH	subcutaneous injection
Lutrepulse	GnRH	subcutaneous injection
Dostinex	Carbergoline	tablet

Risk factors for ovarian cancer may include multiple ovulation and exposure to higher levels of FSH and LH. In fact, most ovarian cancers occur in postmenopausal women with very high levels of FSH and LH. Experts agree, however, that being infertile also is a risk factor for ovarian cancer, especially if a pregnancy is never achieved or carried to term, regardless of whether or not a woman took fertility drugs.

One retrospective study done in 1994 on women who were diagnosed and treated for infertility from 1974 to 1985, indicated that women who take twelve or more cycles of Clomid in a lifetime may increase their overall risk of ovarian cancer when compared with someone who has never taken the drug. Yet a study published in *Fertility and Sterility* in May 1999 revealed no increased risk of breast or ovarian cancer in patients having used fertility drugs. The follow-up time in this study was 17.9 years.

Artificial Insemination

Artificial insemination is the delivery of a partner's or donor's semen into a woman's vagina, cervix, uterus, or fallopian tubes to achieve a pregnancy. This procedure is most useful when the male has a good sperm count and when the woman has anatomical or cervical mucus problems, but it is often used to enhance chances of success with fertility drugs or for unexplained infertility.

This procedure has a long history, with the first recorded attempt dating back to 1780. Because artificial insemination is simple and inexpensive compared to other treatment options, it is the one most couples and physicians turn to first when appropriate. Many women will take fertility drugs prior to insemination. However, insemination success depends on a competent physician first determining through an HSG that a woman's fallopian tubes are clear. Attempts at insemination are futile if sperm cannot get through the tubes to fertilize the egg.

Timing the Insemination

After a patient is determined by a physician to be a good candidate for artificial insemination, the woman is monitored by either ovulation kits, ultrasound, or blood tests throughout the first half of her cycle. Then, when she is ovulating, her partner's sperm are processed and inseminated into her reproductive tract through a catheter. Artificial insemination may also be performed using donor sperm, an option chosen by single women as well as couples with severe male factor infertility.

Most physicians prefer to have the man masturbate, ejaculating into a sterile container at the lab; the sperm is needed for processing within 1 hour of ejaculation. The clinic will either inseminate once or twice in the cycle. Most inseminations are done 24 to 36 hours after an hCG shot or after the ovulation monitoring device shows there has been a hormonal change and that ovulation is pending.

Sperm Preparation

Before it is delivered to the woman's reproductive tract, the sperm is "washed." To accomplish this, once the sperm liquefies at room temperature for about 30 minutes, it is placed in a harmless chemical that isolates the most active sperm. Then it may be "spun" in a machine, a centrifuge, so the best-swimming sperm are collected. This process increases the chance of fertilization because only the healthiest sperm are used. The process also removes various chemicals in the semen that could cause severe cramping if "unwashed" sperm were injected into the uterus.

How Many Inseminations Are Needed?

It may take three to four cycles to achieve a pregnancy through ovulation induction and artificial insemination. Success rates for artificial insemination vary according to both partners' fertility problems, but about 40 percent of women who undergo artificial insemination are pregnant after six attempts. The procedure is performed about 650,000 times a year, with a 15 percent pregnancy success rate for the husband's sperm and a 25 percent success rate for donor sperm. Costs range from $500 to $1,500 per cycle.

Intrauterine Insemination

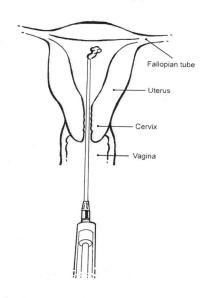

For intrauterine insemination, the sperm is injected into the uterus with a catheter.

A problem with sperm antibodies in the cervical mucus can be treated by bypassing the mucus using *intrauterine insemination*. This involves placing specially prepared sperm into the uterus using a small rubber catheter passed up through the cervical canal at the time of a woman's ovulation.

Reversal of Sterilization

Because medications and IVF are so effective in treating a variety of fertility problems, the only type of microsurgery that is regularly performed is that of "untying" a woman's tubes to reverse sterilization. *Microsurgery* is reconstructive surgery performed under magnification using delicate instruments and precise techniques. Success rates for this particular procedure range from 25 percent to 85 percent, depending on how much healthy tube is available. Having this procedure performed does result in a higher risk of ectopic pregnancy.

Sterilization reversal and the majority of other reproductive surgeries are performed on an outpatient basis. Patients may go home to recuperate the same day or the next and are back at work within three to ten days.

Other Treatments

Other treatments for female infertility include the removal of polyps, fibroids, or endometriosis through a hysteroscopy or laparoscopy, as discussed in chapter 3.

Less commonly, a *laparotomy* is performed. Laparotomy is a major surgery that requires making a large incision in order to better visualize and access the pelvic organs. The procedure may be needed to remove fibroids, occasionally to treat a ruptured ectopic pregnancy, or to treat severe endometriosis that cannot be treated through a laparoscope.

Treatment for Secondary Infertility

Treatment options for patients with secondary infertility are the same as those for patients who have never achieved a full-term pregnancy. However, there is evidence that pregnancy rates are 2 to 12 percent higher in patients with secondary infertility, depending on the age of the female. Unfortunately, those suffering from secondary infertility are only about half as likely to seek treatment, possibly due in part to the difficulties of raising a child while simultaneously struggling to conceive another.

Those with secondary infertility may find emotional support lacking. Friends and family may assume the couple does not desire more children for personal reasons. Or, since the couple already has children, others may not view their desire for another child with empathy and understanding. Although secondary infertility brings with it some different emotional issues, it may be as emotionally painful as primary infertility. Their child's pleas for a sister or brother can make these couples feel guilty and inadequate. Pressure from extended family members for another grandchild may also increase feelings of frustration.

5

Assisted Reproductive Technologies (ARTs)

Diagnosed with moderate endometriosis, Angie elected to try in vitro fertilization after four failed artificial insemination attempts. Ten eggs were retrieved from her ovaries, and six of them fertilized with her husband's sperm. Her doctor decided to transfer three embryos to her uterus and freeze the rest. Ten days later, her pregnancy test was positive, and she was delighted to discover at a subsequent ultrasound that she was expecting twins.

"Going through infertility treatment was one of the most difficult and depressing things I have ever done. I cried a lot and at times was absolutely sure I would never be a mother. I find it amazing that now, just six months after my babies' births, I have trouble recalling all the details of what it took to get them here. Even so, my infertility experience will always be a part of me. I know I wouldn't have them without these advanced technologies, and I feel so fortunate."

What Is ART?

Assisted reproductive technology (ART) includes a number of high-tech treatments in which eggs are removed from a woman's ovary, fertilized outside the body, and then transferred back into her body. ART can be used for women with tubal problems, endometriosis, age-related infertility, and unexplained infertility. ART is also used if there is a severe male factor problem.

In 1981 the first American baby was born as a result of in vitro fertilization, an ART procedure. Since then, ART procedures have been refined. As success rates continue to increase, couples have more reason to hope for a positive outcome.

In Vitro Fertilization

The most common ART is in vitro fertilization (IVF)—a technique that has proven particularly successful for women with blocked or damaged fallopian tubes, men with sperm abnormalities, and for couples with unexplained infertility. IVF involves retrieving a woman's eggs from the ovary and fertilizing them with her husband's or a donor's sperm in the lab. Two to four of the resulting embryos are placed in the uterus to (hopefully) implant. This procedure was initially referred to as producing a "test-tube" baby, but is now commonly known as IVF.

I've been in infertility treatment for seven years and am expecting my first child. My second IVF worked. I've seen four physicians.

Marcie, 34
Diagnosis: endometriosis

The first IVF baby was born in 1978 in England. Since then, more than 35,000 babies have been born through IVF in the United States alone. Once considered a miracle, fertilization outside the body is practiced daily at more than 300 fertility clinics across the country, with 63,814 cycles of IVFs performed in 1999. Most of these clinics have a 30 to up to 45 percent live birth rate per embryo transfer, which is better than that of couples without fertility problems trying on their own in any given month.

A woman's age is the key factor that determines whether she will get pregnant through IVF. The younger a woman is, the higher her probability of becoming pregnant through IVF. The procedure requires frequent monitoring of how the ovaries are responding to stimulation. Cost of the procedure ranges from $5,000 to $15,000 per cycle.

Retrieving and Fertilizing the Eggs

With the help of fertility drugs, many women produce several eggs during a given cycle—anywhere from two to twenty or more. Because there is a risk of multiple gestations with IVF, physicians determine how many embryos to place in a woman's uterus based on her age, embryo quality, and other health factors.

Once the follicles appear to be mature, based on blood tests and an ultrasound test, they are retrieved. To accomplish this, a needle is used to aspirate, or remove, the eggs from the ovary. Intravenous sedation is usually used, and the egg retrieval is typically completed in less than 30 minutes.

On the day of the egg retrieval, the sperm sample is processed to recover the healthiest sperm; the sperm may come from a partner who provides the sample through masturbation or the sperm may have been donated. An embryologist, a specialist in embryo development, inspects the eggs and allows them to incubate in *culture media*, a fluid with the necessary ingredients for proper cell growth outside the body. Close attention is paid to the laboratory environment so that the sperm, egg, and eventual embryo can grow optimally. After a few hours, the sperm are mixed with, or injected into, the mature eggs and incubated overnight. The next morning, the eggs are checked for fertilization.

Three days later, after the sperm and egg have grown from a single-cell embryo to an eight-cell embryo, selected fertilized embryos are transferred. They are transferred to the uterus using a tiny catheter and sometimes with the guidance of ultrasound. Most women experience no discomfort. Some say it feels much like an intrauterine insemination.

Ensuring Implantation

As techniques have been refined, it has been determined that some women may have much better implantation rates if the embryos are cultured longer to the *blastocyst stage*. The blastocyst stage is the stage at which the embryo is normally capable of implantation—about five days after the egg is retrieved from the woman's ovary. Prior to 1999, when this technique was pioneered, embryos were transferred on day two or three. But the development of a new type of amino acid-based culture fluid now allows embryos to live in the laboratory for five days or more—until they reach their full maturity at the blastocyst stage.

I always remained positive. I just kept thinking that I could get pregnant. I was aware of all the technology that could help us, and finally it did.

Sue, 35
expecting a baby
Diagnosis: endometriosis

The embryologist can usually choose the best embryos for transfer. High-quality blastocyst embryos are more likely to implant, fewer embryos need to be transferred and the risk of multiple gestations is diminished. Pregnancy rates, however, do not appear to be higher. To increase the likelihood of implantation, some patients may benefit from *assisted hatching* on the embryos before transfer to the uterus. In this procedure, a tiny opening is made in the *zona*, or outer wall, of the embryo using a laser or a special chemical. The theory is that by making an opening in the embryo wall, the embryo will be better able to attach to the uterine wall and burrow in more easily. Still, this procedure does not benefit all patients and is best used selectively. The risks of this procedure include damage to the embryo and increased risk of having identical twins.

Some clinics use low doses of steroids and antibiotics with embryo transfer to prevent infections from developing; however, this has not been scientifically proven to be of benefit.

After IVF

Most physicians prescribe progesterone after embryo transfer to assist with endometrial development and as a precaution against miscarriage. This medication is taken orally, vaginally, or by intramuscular injection. A blood pregnancy test can be taken about ten days after embryo transfer.

Intracytoplasmic Sperm Injection (ICSI)

Another newer technique used in conjunction with IVF is *intracytoplasmic sperm injection (ICSI)*. In contrast to standard IVF, where the eggs are placed in the same dish with the sperm and allowed to fertilize, ICSI involves the direct injection of a single sperm into a single egg to achieve fertilization.

The first child conceived through ICSI was born in the United States in 1993. ICSI has greatly increased fertilization rates and has even been called the "solution" to male-factor fertilization problems. In some programs, ICSI will add approximately $2,000 to $4,000 to the cost of IVF. As with standard IVF, there does not appear to be a higher incidence of birth defects in children conceived through ICSI, although there are some concerns. For example, it has been found that some male factor infertility is inherited. It is possible for men with no sperm or severely low sperm counts to pass these genetic abnormalities on to their male offspring.

Genetic testing and counseling should be offered to all patients considering ICSI for severe male factor infertility. As with standard IVF, the age of the female partner is a key factor that determines whether the procedure will be a success. ICSI success is also dependent on the skill of the embryologist who is preparing the sperm and the egg and inserting the one sperm into the egg. Therefore, it is important that patients make sure that the clinic they are considering is experienced with ICSI.

I was ready to do all I could to get pregnant. My third in vitro attempt was successful. We used a donor egg, and we have a beautiful son.

Jean, 27
Diagnosis: small ovary and no fallopian tube

Multiple Births

Because multiple embryos are generated and transferred in IVF cycles, there is a risk of multiple gestation. The resulting multiple births increase the risk of injury to mother and babies and are considered the greatest potential hazard of medically assisted reproduction. See chapter 9 for more information on multiple births.

Other ART Procedures

Gamete Intrafallopian Transfer (GIFT)

For this procedure, eggs are first taken from the ovary. Then the eggs and sperm are placed directly into the fallopian tubes in an effort to mimic nature more closely. The procedure also involves the use of follicle-stimulating drugs and sperm-washing techniques. GIFT is not performed as much nowadays since the physician cannot tell if fertilization has occurred, and the procedure requires a laparoscopy and general anesthesia.

Zygote Intrafallopian Transfer (ZIFT)

ZIFT also involves the use of follicle-stimulating drugs, egg retrieval, and sperm-washing techniques. However, it is different from GIFT in that the eggs are fertilized in the laboratory before they are placed in the woman's fallopian tube. ZIFT has the advantage of allowing the physician to confirm fertilization before transferring the eggs. The embryo transfer is made more quickly than with IVF, usually within a day or two. If all goes well, the embryo develops in the tube for several more days while the uterus readies itself for implantation. Then it moves naturally into place.

In some cases, low-grade embryos may do better in the fallopian tubes than in the uterus. However, use of the ZIFT procedure is declining because it is more expensive and more invasive, with no better success rates than IVF.

Both ZIFT and GIFT are used much less frequently than IVF. In 1999, the number of IVF procedures performed in the United States was 63,814. That compares to 868 GIFT and 1,302 ZIFT procedures.

Choosing an ART Clinic

Because the booming infertility industry is largely unregulated, patients must be careful in selecting a clinic for assisted reproductive technology. Find out if the staff is affiliated with a major academic medical center, and ask about the credentials and training of the physicians. It's also important to ascertain whether the physicians are active members of the Society for Reproductive Endocrinology and Infertility or the American Society for Reproductive Medicine. Both are respected professional organizations.

Information on clinic success rates is available from the Centers for Disease Control's ART clinic success rate report, which is published every year. Under federal law, all ART clinics are required to report their statistics on birth rates for a variety of age categories, as well as for frozen embryo transfers. This report is available free through the Centers for Disease Control (CDC) by mail or on-line at www.cdc.gov.

My two cousins and two friends have all offered to have a child for us. It means a lot to me that they offered, but my husband is not in favor of this option.

Chris, 33
Diagnosis: unexplained infertility

When looking at a clinic's success rates, make certain you understand their statistics. Reporting styles for pregnancy rates differ from clinic to clinic and can be misleading to the average consumer. For example, some doctors will perform IVF on a couple only twice and don't accept patients over age 40. As a result, their patients are younger and achieve success more easily. Accordingly, their success rates are high.

When considering a fertility clinic, ask the physician or staff the following questions:

- Does the clinic accept everyone? Is there a limit on the number of times a procedure is performed?
- Will the clinic work with women over age 40 or those with an elevated day-3 FSH blood level? Does the clinic have a donor egg program?
- If you're not responding well to the treatment, will the clinic drop you or keep trying?
- What is the doctor's cancellation rate per cycle?
- When did the clinic start offering ART? How many patients undergo IVF each year? Clinics who have been doing ART procedures for many years may have the best results.
- What is the clinic's delivery rate per treatment cycle initiated for women in your age category? Also ask about the number of miscarriages, live births, and multiple births relative to the number of embryo transfers.
- Does the clinic freeze extra embryos? If so, what is the viability rate of those embryos after thawing?
- What does each cycle cost, including drugs and ultrasounds? Is payment expected up front?

It's also important to be mindful of false advertising. Since 1991, the Federal Trade Commission has obtained cease and desist orders against eleven clinics who falsely advertised quick and easy ways to achieve a pregnancy. Although the majority of clinics are reputable, it still pays to do a little research before placing your personal health, finances, and hopes for a child in the hands of any physician.

6

Donor Eggs and Donor Sperm

Mary and Ted knew when they got married that they would need help achieving a pregnancy. Ted had been diagnosed with testicular cancer at age 22 and had undergone chemotherapy. Before taking chemotherapy, his doctors urged him to freeze some sperm for later use, but Ted, frightened and consumed by his illness, had resisted their urgings and not given it much thought until he'd met Mary.

When fertility tests determined Ted was not producing sperm, the couple decided to pursue sperm donation. "We were both comfortable with it but worried about what other people might think, so we decided not to tell anyone we used a donor," Mary says. "We just didn't want everyone gossiping about us and labeling our child. Now we just smile when family members say how much our son looks like Ted. It took some getting used to, but I really don't think it bothers Ted at all now. He's our son, and that's all there is to it. We plan to tell our son the truth about his conception when he's older, and we are using the same donor for our next baby."

Using Donor Eggs

Egg donation involves retrieving eggs from a donor's ovaries, fertilizing them with sperm from either the infertile woman's partner or a donor, and transferring the fertilized embryo into the infertile woman's uterus. Any embryos not used in the initial procedure can be frozen for later use, making it possible for a family to have genetically-related children.

Egg donation can come from anonymous or known sources. Generally, donor eggs are difficult to obtain, so many women use a sister's or a friend's eggs. Even if egg donors are known, they should be screened in the same manner as anonymous donors. If an anonymous donor's eggs are used, most physicians try to match the donor's and patient's physical characteristics, such as blood type and hair and eye color.

We have two children conceived with donor sperm. I felt my husband needed to feel totally comfortable about using donor sperm. I was afraid he might have second thoughts later on.
Karen, 36
Diagnosis: male factor and blocked tubes

Some clinics use college students as donors because their youth generally makes them more fertile. Some consider this practice controversial because young women may be risking their own future fertility by taking fertility drugs and donating their eggs. Some clinics require donors to have had healthy children of their own and have no plans for more.

High Success Rates

Egg donation has made it possible for women to become pregnant at almost any age. In fact, donor egg pregnancy rates for older women, those over 40, are as high as 60 to 70 percent, making it an important option for younger women who have diseased or absent ovaries or are experiencing early menopause.

In 1994, in Italy, a 62-year-old woman gave birth to a baby conceived with donor eggs and her husband's sperm. Although births by postmenopausal women are controversial and rare, they underscore the astonishing medical advancements being made in the fertility industry.

Costs for IVF with Donated Eggs

The costs for IVF with egg donation range from $7,000 to more than $20,000. Clinics that split a donor's eggs between two patients can offer cost savings and a shorter wait to receive them.

We tried every new procedure, and finally decided to use donor sperm and eggs, but we didn't tell our families. Now that I am pregnant, family members talk about who the babies will look like. It's hard to deal with these remarks.

Cathy, 34, expecting twins Diagnosis: unexplained infertility

Using Donor Sperm

Sperm donation involves the storage and use of an anonymous man's sperm with either an artificial insemination or IVF procedure. Success rates are high with donor sperm because this sperm has been screened for sperm count, motility (motion), and morphology (shape). The sperm is also carefully screened for health risks such as chromosomal abnormalities, sexually transmitted diseases, HIV, hepatitis, and cystic fibrosis.

Most sperm banks will provide information to the patient about the sperm donor's hair and eye color, ethnicity, health history, and education. In turn, this information should be made available to the patient or couple.

Women with no known fertility problems who choose donor insemination will normally achieve a pregnancy in three to four cycles. Using donor sperm is relatively inexpensive—about $500 to $700 per cycle.

Making the Decision

Choosing to use donor eggs or sperm is difficult for most couples. They may view it as not being able to have children who are their own "flesh and blood." This means giving up part of the dream of reproducing with their own genes and having a child that is part of each of them. It is important to grieve that loss before moving on to using donor eggs or sperm.

For some couples, using donor eggs or sperm is their only chance of having a partially biological child. Couples must examine their feelings honestly, and should receive counseling prior to making a decision.

7

Male Factor Infertility

David and Mary were surprised to discover that David's sperm analysis showed he had a low sperm count. After considering their options, they decided to undergo in vitro fertilization (IVF) and Mary became pregnant.

Looking back, David realizes that he was embarrassed about his diagnosis and didn't want anyone to know about it. But since then, he has had a change of heart and willingly shares his story with other men experiencing male factor infertility. "I found that the more open I was about my diagnosis, the more comfortable and hopeful I felt that we would have a baby of our own one day. I told my doctor to refer other men to me if they'd like to talk to someone who has gone through this difficult experience."

Coping Emotionally

Historically, infertility has been viewed as a female problem, rather than a male one. A diagnosis of male infertility leaves many men feeling ashamed and embarrassed, mostly because they mistakenly equate fertility with virility. A man may also worry that others will find out about his infertility and assume he is not "man enough" to produce a child. The fact is, sexual dysfunction in the infertile man is rare, so virility and fertility are two separate issues.

Still, a man's self-image and emotional well-being may be affected, and so may the couple's sexual relationship. Accordingly, open communication between the couple is key to keeping a healthy perspective on the matter. Keep in mind that no one is to blame for infertility. Infertility is a shared experience, and the emotional and physical health of each individual relies on a united approach. In the end, many men say working together with their female partners to overcome their infertility makes them stronger and closer as a couple. Some men find it helpful to seek out support from groups. Others may wish to find a Web site that provides anonymous information and support.

As a man goes through the process of being diagnosed with a fertility problem, it is important to note that 50 percent of male infertility problems are treatable.

Risk Factors for Male Infertility

Injury

Injury or trauma resulting from such things as sporting accidents or motor vehicle crashes can impair a man's ability to produce sperm. Injuries may include damage to the testicles or rupture or tearing of the *vas deferens*, a delicate tube that carries the sperm from the testicle to the ejaculatory duct. Damage to other parts of the body, including the prostate gland or bladder, may also affect sperm production. Spinal cord injuries may effect ejaculation and semen delivery, resulting in male infertility.

Male Reproductive System

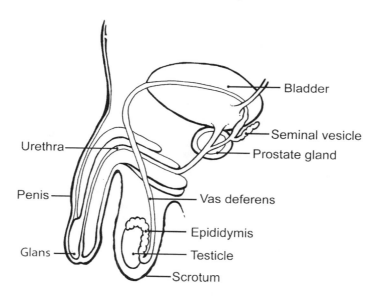

Testicular torsion, a condition caused by the testicles twisting inside the scrotum, can also lead to infertility. Each testicle, or *testis,* is suspended from *spermatic cords* within the scrotum. These cords carry sperm from the testicles and also supply blood to them. A twisting of the testicle and cords pinches off the blood supply. The loss of blood causes tissue damage to the testicle.

If surgery is performed to untwist the testicle within twelve hours after the onset of symptoms, the testicle can be saved in about 70 percent of cases. Delayed treatment often results in damage to the testicle, seriously impairing fertility. Torsion occurs more frequently in adolescents. This painful injury most frequently occurs at night or in the early morning when a young man is asleep. Symptoms include sudden, severe pain and swelling.

Sexually Transmitted Diseases (STDs)

Sexually transmitted diseases (STDs) are often related to male infertility. For example, if left untreated, the STD chlamydia can lead to scarring of the urethra, which carries semen through the penis. Such scarring can obstruct the flow of semen. Often, a man does not know he has chlamydia. In fact, one out of two men doesn't get early symptoms. Those who do have symptoms experience a discharge from the penis, a burning sensation during urination, or swollen testicles.

At first, I had a hard time accepting that my sperm was inadequate. Finally I realized it was not my fault and that I wasn't the only one with the problem. My wife was very supportive.
John, 27
Diagnosis: low sperm count

Smoking

Like women, men may be affected by cigarette smoking when it comes to fertility. According to the journal *Fertility and Sterility,* studies show male smokers may have more abnormally shaped sperm and sperm with genetic defects when compared with nonsmoking men. Although smoking may not make a man infertile, it may be a factor in a man whose sperm count is already compromised.

Substance Abuse

Abuse of drugs and alcohol may cause infertility in a man. Chronic alcoholism that results in liver damage may result in infertility. Also, smoking marijuana may affect fertility by causing reduced LH secretions and reduced production of testosterone. A reduction in testosterone may lead to impotence and lower sperm counts. Also, many body-building drugs cause a reduction in LH and testosterone, ultimately shrinking the size of the testicles.

Excessive Heat

High heat such as that in hot tubs, whirlpools, and saunas may also affect a man's fertility. Since the testicles and sperm production are affected by high heat, men may wish to avoid these settings if they're at risk for infertility and intend to conceive with a mate.

Stress

Stress is a factor in all functions of male health and wellness. Stress may interfere with the LH that controls testicular function. This may lead to a reduction in sperm count or an impairment in sperm function.

Exposure to DES

If a man was exposed to the drug diethylstilbestrol (DES) while in his mother's uterus, the formation of his reproductive system, including the sperm ducts and testicles, may have been impaired. In turn, his sperm production may be affected.

Environmental Factors

Exposure to chemicals or toxins may have an effect on male fertility. Some pesticides and herbicides, which have estrogen-like effects, could impair sperm production. Other chemicals that may have an impact on male fertility include heavy metals such as lead, cadmium, and arsenic.

Causes of Male Infertility

Since approximately half of all infertility problems can be attributed in some way to the male, it is important that the male be tested along with the female. There are a variety of causes for male infertility; however, the most common are related to sperm production and maturation and obstructions in the tubes that carry sperm.

Sperm Abnormality

The amount of sperm a man has in his ejaculate and the quality of the sperm are the key factors in male fertility. Problems arise if the volume of semen is low, the sperm count is low, or the sperm are unable to move properly. A low sperm count is referred to as *oligospermia*. In some men, sperm production is absent. If a man has no sperm, the condition is known as *azoospermia*. In many cases, the exact causes of sperm abnormality cannot be determined.

Varicoceles

About 15 percent of men are estimated to have *varicoceles*, a collection of varicose veins in the scrotum. Approximately 40 percent of men with varicoceles have fertility problems, making varicoceles a common cause of male infertility. A varicocele develops because of defective valves that normally allow blood to flow away from the testicles toward the abdomen. Instead, the blood pools, and the veins become dilated or enlarged.

It's not fully understood how varicoceles affect sperm production, but the main theory is that the dilated blood vessels of a varicocele raise the temperature around the testicles. An increase in heat of even one degree can have an adverse effect on the ability of the testicles to produce sperm normally.

Although they are more common on the left side, varicoceles may appear on both sides of the scrotum. Rarely do they appear on the right side only. During an examination, a physician can feel varicoceles that would impair fertility.

Varicocele

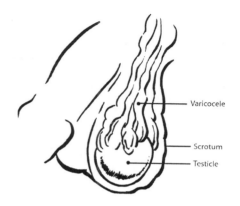

A collection of blood vessels in the scrotum, a varicocele is usually found on the left side.

Damage to the Duct System

One of the most common obstructions to the duct system, which transports sperm, results from a voluntary *vasectomy* that a man later wishes to have reversed. A popular method of birth control, a vasectomy sterilizes a man by clipping the tubes that carry sperm. An estimated 500,000 to 1 million men have vasectomies annually in the United States, and the demand for vasectomy reversal is on the rise.

Aside from vasectomy reversal, it's estimated that 7 to 9 percent of infertile men have blockages in the network of delicate ducts that carry sperm. These ducts include the *epididymis*, vas deferens, and ejaculatory ducts. Such blockages may occur anywhere in the duct system between the testicles and the urethra. The blockages may have been present at birth, or the ductal damage may have occurred later in the man's life. He may have damage resulting from a previous surgery, such as a hernia repair, in which the vas deferens or the blood supply to the testicles was affected. This damage may result in reduced sperm counts or even a total blockage of sperm production.

Genetic and Congenital Disorders

In some men, parts of the reproductive system may be malformed or missing. For example, approximately 1 percent of men are born with an *undescended testicle*, one that never descended into the scrotum. If left untreated, the testicle function is impaired. Surgery to bring the testicle down is recommended during infancy, preferably before the age of two. An undescended testicle does not necessarily mean a man will be infertile, but the condition is a clear risk factor for male infertility.

Approximately 1 percent of men are born without a *vas deferens*. A missing vas deferens may also be a symptom of another potential problem—men without a vas deferens on both sides may carry a gene that causes cystic fibrosis, a serious disease that causes the body to produce abnormal amounts of sticky mucus in the lining of the lungs and pancreas. These men should be screened for cystic fibrosis before proceeding with any form of fertility treatment since this trait can be passed on to children if the man's sperm is used.

Research shows a man's sperm count may be the result of genetics. In men with severely low sperm counts, there is a 3 to 6 percent chance that an abnormality of the Y chromosome is present. This abnormality can be passed on to male offspring. An abnormality of the Y chromosome has also been found in approximately 20 percent of males with no sperm in their specimen. This abnormality will also be passed to male offspring.

Other genetic disorders also affect fertility. *Klinefelter's syndrome*, a condition in which an extra X chromosome is present, may lead to male infertility. The symptoms of this syndrome are small testicles and occasionally enlarged breasts. Klinefelter's syndrome is diagnosed through a chromosome analysis.

Another cause of male infertility is *Sertoli cell only syndrome*, a rare condition in which sperm-producing cells in the testicles did not develop during fetal development. Sertoli cells actively control sperm production in the testicles, but when sperm is absent a man is said to have "Sertoli cells only." This condition may be congenital or may result from other life events such as radiation or chemotherapy, which may destroy sperm-producing cells.

We didn't know about my husband's infertility until three months into my own treatment. When we realized his problem was severe, we also began looking into adoption and using donor sperm.

Stephanie, 34
Diagnosis: polycystic ovary syndrome and male factor

Immunologic Disorders

As mentioned in chapter 2, immunologic disorders such as sperm antibodies result from the body attacking its own cells as if they were foreign materials or bacteria. Approximately 10 percent of infertile men are found to have such antibodies. The cause for sperm antibodies is not clear; however, physicians believe a number of conditions may influence their formation. These include chemotherapy, exposure to pesticides, vasectomy reversal, trauma, testicular torsion, testicular cancer, infections, and hernia repair.

Antibodies on the sperm's head are the primary cause of immunologic infertility. These antibodies can impair the sperm's ability to penetrate an egg. A lab can determine whether antibodies are present by examining a semen sample. If a semen analysis shows that the sperm *agglutinate*, or clump together, antibodies are suspected.

Also, up to 70 percent of men who have had vasectomy reversals are found to have sperm antibodies. The antibodies are believed to form after a vasectomy when the sperm, which can no longer be ejaculated, leak out into the body. The immune system treats them as foreign material and antibodies develop.

Infections

Infections can play a role in male infertility. These inflammations may create scarring that blocks the tubes that carry sperm, or they may affect sperm production or movement. These infections include:

- *Prostatitis*: Infection of the prostate gland.
- *Epididymitis*: Infection of the epididymis, a tube that helps carry sperm from the testicles.
- *Orchitis*: Inflammation of the testicles.
- *Urethritis*: Inflammation of the urethra, the tube that carries both urine and sperm through the penis.
- *Cystitis*: Inflammation of the bladder.
- *Mumps*: Occurring after puberty, the mumps virus can enter the testicles, impairing the ability to produce

sperm. About 25 percent of men who've had mumps after puberty have damage to their testicles.

Pituitary Hormone Deficiencies

Hormonal deficiencies of the pituitary gland are not a common cause of infertility in men. It's estimated that approximately 2 percent of male infertility cases result from abnormal hormone levels of pituitary hormones. The condition *hypogonadotropic hypogonadism* results from men having low levels of the gonadotropins FSH and LH. In women, these hormones affect ovulation. In men, they influence the production of the male hormone testosterone, which in turn affects sperm production.

Ejaculatory Problems

Ejaculation is the emission of semen from the penis. Common reasons for lack of ejaculation include impotency and retrograde ejaculation.

Impotency, the inability to achieve an erection, may be the result of psychological or physical problems. Psychological problems may include anxiety about performing sex, guilt, or low self-esteem. Physical problems that can impair a man's ability to become erect include such diseases as diabetes, high cholesterol, high blood pressure, and heart disease, and the side effects of some medications, including some antidepressants.

Retrograde ejaculation is a condition in which the semen is thrust "backwards" into the bladder instead of being released through the penis during orgasm. Testing for it requires having a man urinate after he ejaculates. Retrograde ejaculation, which is estimated to affect up to 2 percent of infertile men, is likely caused by a weakening of the nerves in the muscle that should close the bladder neck during orgasm. When the bladder neck does not close properly, semen is propelled into the bladder. Men with spinal cord injury, diabetes, multiple sclerosis, previous prostate surgery, and men on some medications (especially those for high blood pressure) may have retrograde ejaculation.

Medications

A number of common medications may affect a man's fertility. The chemical mechanism causing the infertility is complex, but essentially, some drugs may affect the hormones related to sperm production. These drugs include:

- Ketoconazole: an antifungal
- Sulfasalazine: for inflammatory bowel disease
- Spironolactone: an antihypertensive
- Calcium channel blockers: antihypertensives
- Allopurinal, colchicine: for gout
- Nitrofurantoin, erythromycin, gentamicin: antibiotics
- Methotrexate: for cancer, psoriasis, arthritis
- Cimetidine: for ulcers or reflux

Drugs that may cause ejaculatory dysfunction include:

- Antipsychotics: chlorpromazine, haloperidol, thioridazine
- Antidepressants: amitriptyline, imipramine, fluoxetine (Prozac), paroxetine (Paxil), sertraline (Zoloft)
- Antihypertensives: guanethidine, prazosin, phenoxybenzamine, phentolamine, reserpine, thiazides

One class of drugs known to severely impact sperm production are anabolic steroids, sometimes abused by athletes and weight lifters. In some cases, the suppression of male hormones caused by anabolic steroids may be permanent.

Getting a Diagnosis

The Initial Examination

In many cases, a man will first be examined by his primary care physician. The physician will usually order a semen analysis to determine whether a problem exists with sperm production; if the analysis shows an abnormality, the primary care physician will often refer the man to a urologist. Other times, the physician treating a man's female partner will order the semen analysis. The woman's physician will also likely refer the man to a urologist if a problem is found. A *urologist* is a physician who specializes in disorders of the kidneys, urinary tract, bladder, and male reproductive organs.

Once referred to a urologist, a man will undergo a thorough physical examination and an extensive medical history will be taken. Most men are asked to answer a lengthy questionnaire that includes questions about:

- duration of unprotected intercourse
- nature and volume of his ejaculate
- history of fathering other children
- injuries or trauma to the genitals
- illnesses, including mumps
- infections, including sexually transmitted diseases
- past surgeries
- undescended testicles

- current medications
- environmental factors—stress, smoking, or alcohol/drug use

During the physical examination, the physician will likely draw a blood sample, which will usually be tested for infections and hormone levels. The physician will carefully examine the genitals. Testicles and the networks of tubes surrounding them are checked for size and location. Urine and semen samples may also be collected.

Although an abundance of high technology is available, most urologists report that they can frequently make a diagnosis after a patient's initial visit, based on his medical history, physical exam, and semen test.

The Semen Analysis

The *semen analysis* is one of the fundamental tests performed to determine male infertility. This test determines whether a man is producing sperm of a quality that will impregnate a female. A basic semen analysis examines the sperm volume, movement, and number, all of which may affect fertility. These factors are determined by a microscopic examination of a sperm sample.

Collecting the Semen

When a man is producing a semen specimen for examination, it is considered optimal that he abstain from ejaculating for a period of 2 to 5 days before the specimen is collected. If the specimen is collected without a period of abstinence, the number of sperm in his ejaculate may be reduced. And, if he waits longer than 5 days, the prolonged abstinence may affect

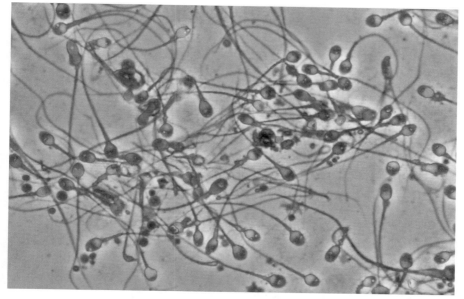

Human sperm magnified one thousand times. *Photo by Michael Howell.*

the sperm's ability to move. Either of these situations could influence the results of the semen analysis. So, for the most accurate results, 3 to 5 days of abstinence are recommended. If abnormal results are discovered in the analysis, two to three analyses should be done.

To collect a sample, men are usually asked to go to a physician's clinic where they masturbate, catching the total ejaculate in a sterile container. Obtaining the specimen on-site ensures that it is delivered to the lab in a timely manner, that its temperature remains constant, and that it is not exposed to outside elements.

Some clinics allow men to collect the sample at home and take it directly to the lab. If the specimen is produced at home, it must be kept at body temperature and evaluated at the lab within an hour of collection. Men whose religious beliefs preclude them from masturbating can wear a special collection condom during intercourse and deliver an adequate specimen for evaluation. Ordinary rubber condoms won't work since they usually contain powders or spermicides that would damage the sperm sample.

Evaluating the Sperm

Sperm Volume

The sperm sample is first evaluated for volume. The volume of sperm in a normal ejaculate is 2 to 5 milliliters, or about a teaspoon. A large ejaculate, however, is not an indication of fertility. For example, a man's ejaculate may be double the normal size, yet he could be infertile.

Sperm Count

The number of sperm in the ejaculate is critical to conception. A sperm count is expressed as the number of million sperm per milliliter. A sperm count is considered adequate if it is greater than 20 million per milliliter. A sperm count below 10 million can have a negative impact on fertilization. Sperm densities below 1 million represent severe male factor infertility. Spontaneous fertilization through intercourse will most likely not occur under these conditions.

Men's fertility does not appear to dramatically change with age. Studies do report a slight drop in the count and quality of sperm when men reach their 50s, but reproductive changes in men are far less dramatic and more gradual than those in women.

Liquefaction

Initially, upon ejaculation, semen coagulates. Then, over the course of 30 to 60 minutes, it will liquefy. Liquefaction is important because if the semen does not go through this process, the sperm will not be able to swim through the cervical mucus and into the uterus.

Morphology

Sperm morphology refers to its shape. It is unclear whether the overall sperm shape affects sperm function. Some sperm with two heads, two tails, or bizarre shape are unlikely to penetrate the egg, but most fertile men's semen contains a large variety of sperm shapes. Many studies show no connection between the average sperm shape of a man and his chances for conceiving a child.

Motility

Motility refers to whether the sperm is motile, or moving. Fifty percent or more of the sperm should show movement. *Forward progression* refers to the extent to which the sperm are moving forward. It is generally believed that sperm with forward progression has a better chance to fertilize an egg.

Treatments for Male Infertility

Surgery for Varicoceles

Surgical repair of a significant varicocele is performed to eliminate the varicose veins around the testicles. Surgical treatment offers the best results. Semen improvement is expected in up to 66 percent of men and pregnancy in up to 43 percent of couples within the first two years after successful repair.

To perform this procedure with conventional surgery, the physician makes a three-inch or smaller incision in the groin, lifts the spermatic cords out of the scrotum, and ties off the enlarged veins attached to the cords. Tying off the veins does not affect blood flow to the testicles. This surgery is usually done on an outpatient basis while a patient is under general anesthesia. It does require a few weeks for full recovery.

Microsurgery can also be used to treat a varicocele. In microsurgery, tiny instruments are used and the surgery is done using a microscope. Microsurgery is also an outpatient procedure, and advantages include a smaller incision, a lower varicocele recurrence rate, and a shorter recovery time. The procedure also protects the arteries supplying blood to the testicles.

Another outpatient procedure, a *balloon occlusion*, is performed with the patient under light sedation. The balloon occlusion involves making a tiny incision in the groin and threading a tiny tube into the vein that is causing the varicocele. The tube is then inflated or "ballooned" to block off the portion of the vein that is defective. This action does not impede blood flow to the testicles.

Although these surgical repairs may be helpful, men also have nonsurgical options. A man and his partner may choose to have intracytoplasmic sperm injection (ICSI), in which a single sperm is used to fertilize a single egg. Another factor to consider is the age of the man's female partner. If her egg quality is diminishing already, the couple may wish to avoid any delay resulting from surgery and move forward with ICSI.

Repairing Ductal Damage

The most common duct repair is a vasectomy reversal. Here, the physician cuts away the blocked area created by the vasectomy and reconnects the tubes with the help of a microscope. Urologic surgeons report success rates, as defined by the presence of sperm in the semen, up to 90 percent if less than 10 years have passed since the vasectomy was performed. Those who wait more than 10 years to pursue reversal face much lower success rates. These men may require IVF with intracytoplasmic sperm injection (ICSI) to achieve pregnancy with their mates.

A man may also be born with, or later develop, blockage of the ducts in the scrotum. In some cases, surgery may remove blockages from these ducts, allowing sperm to travel though them. If surgery is unsuccessful, sperm may be obtained directly from a testicle for use in IVF with ICSI. Or, if a man wishes to avoid surgery, he and his partner may wish to consider IVF with ICSI. If cost is a factor in making a decision, reconstructive surgery is usually not as expensive as IVF; however, it may not be as successful.

Testicular Needle Aspiration

A physician performs a *testicular needle aspiration* to retrieve sperm directly from a man's testicle. The physician inserts a thin needle into the testicle to draw out the sperm. If healthy sperm cells are found inside the testicle, it is possible to extract them and use them fresh or freeze them for future use with ICSI. Testicular needle aspiration is often used for men with severe infertility factor caused by either poor sperm production or a blockage in the duct system that cannot be surgically repaired. A needle aspiration is an office procedure that can be performed in a doctor's office with local anesthesia.

Testicular Biopsy

Another way to obtain sperm directly from a testicle is *testicular biopsy*. This procedure may be performed in an outpatient operating room, often under local anesthesia. A small incision is made in the scrotum, and a sample of tissue is taken for microscopic evaluation and processing. Often used with ICSI, the sperm from the testicular tissue is placed directly into a woman's egg.

When we found out my husband had cancer, we had some of his sperm stored. Later, we tried to conceive. It made me sad to tell him when my period came. He felt it was his fault.
Joy, 29
Diagnosis: irregular cycle and male factor

Testicular biopsy was once more popular solely as a diagnostic tool to determine whether a testicle was producing sperm. Today, however, with advanced reproductive technologies, a biopsy sample will often be sent directly to an embryologist, who will determine whether the tissue contains sperm. If so, the sperm will be used to fertilize the eggs of the female partner.

Whether to have a testicular biopsy or an aspiration is a patient and doctor's preference. Advantages of a testicular biopsy are that small bleeding may be directly controlled, and that more sperm is obtained, especially in cases where sperm production is low. The advantage of a needle aspiration is that it can be performed in a doctor's office, rather than in an outpatient operating room.

Hormone Treatment

Men with abnormal hormone levels may be treated with the same fertility drugs taken by women: clomiphene, hMG (human menopausal gonadotropins), and hCG (human chorionic gonadotropins).

Men with low motility and poor sperm counts due to abnormal hormone levels may benefit from daily doses of clomiphene. Because a sperm requires three months to be produced in the testicles, clomiphene treatment usually requires at least three months for an effect to occur. Occasional side effects of this treatment can include blurred vision and slight breast enlargement or tenderness.

Human chorionic gonadotropins (hCG) and FSH may be required for men with more severe hormonal problems. These are injectable medications that, like clomiphene, must be taken for three months.

Treatment for Retrograde Ejaculation

Over-the-counter *pseudoephedrine* is often used to treat retrograde ejaculation. The brand name for this drug is Sudafed; it is often used for symptoms associated with the common cold. It increases the muscular tone of the bladder neck. If pseudo-ephedrine is not successful, semen may be separated from the urine. If the man is able to urinate, the semen may be retrieved from his urine. If he is unable to urinate, a catheter is inserted through the urethra into the bladder and the semen and urine are drained into a container. In either case, the urine is spun in a centrifuge; the separated semen is then ready for insemination.

Treatment for Immunologic Disorders

It is possible to use *corticosteroids* to treat a man for sperm antibodies; however, this approach may not be successful. These steroids may suppress the immune system and also decrease the formation of antibodies; therapy usually involves taking the steroids for a minimum of one month. Other treatment options include insemination, in which sperm is delivered to the uterus, eliminating the need for the sperm to swim through the cervical mucus. IVF with ICSI—injecting sperm directly into the egg—is considered the most effective treatment for men with high levels of sperm antibodies. Corticosteroids are occasionally used in combination with insemination or IVF with ISCI for the highest chance of success.

Treatment for Ejaculatory Dysfunction

For men who have ejaculatory dysfunction, ejaculation can be induced, usually with vibratory stimulation of the penis or electroejaculation (controlled electrical stimulation). These techniques may be used in men who have suffered a spinal cord injury and are left unable to ejaculate. The date on which these procedures are performed should coincide with ovulation in the female partner.

With vibratory stimulation, a vibrator is placed along the underside of a man's penis, just under the glans, and is turned on and off until the man ejaculates.

Electroejaculation is sometimes performed when vibratory stimulation fails. This procedure is normally performed on a patient under general anesthesia; however, a man with a spinal cord injury may not require anesthesia. To complete the procedure, a probe with electrodes is introduced gently into the rectum. The probe is positioned against the rectal wall at the level of the seminal vesicles and prostate, and the stimulation begins. In 90 percent of cases, sperm can be acquired with this procedure. The sperm may then be used for insemination.

Some physicians will recommend a needle aspiration to retrieve sperm from a testicle, rather than perform electro-ejaculation. With the needle aspiration, IVF with ICSI is needed to achieve a pregnancy.

Insemination or Use of Donor Sperm

If a man's sperm is considered insufficient to cause a pregnancy through intercourse, his physician may consider insemination using his sperm. To improve chances of fertil-ization, the sperm is delivered either to the cervical opening—*cervical insemination*—or into the woman's uterus—*intrauterine insemination.* The sperm is "washed," or processed, to remove the potentially toxic substances in the semen that would cause cramping or infection in the woman.

In other cases, couples with severe male factor infertility may decide to use donor sperm, called *donor insemination* or *DI,* to achieve a pregnancy. DI has a high pregnancy success rate—about 75 percent—as long as the woman has no fertility problems and is younger than age 35. Most couples select an anonymous donor from a professional sperm bank. The woman is inseminated at the time of her ovulation. The couple can choose to buy an extra supply of the donor sperm and freeze it for use in future cycles so that future children would be genetically linked by the same donor. As mentioned in chapter 6, the decision to have DI involves a thorough discussion by the couple, and both partners need to be comfortable with this option.

ARTs for Male Factor Infertility

In years past, severe male factor infertility was often untreatable, and insemination with donor sperm was frequently the only option available to couples. However, in the past decade, new assisted reproductive technologies (ARTs) have made effective treatments possible for thousands of patients. The most popular technique is ICSI, discussed in chapter 5. This procedure involves inserting one sperm into an egg during the IVF procedure.

8

Emotional Impact of Infertility

After each failed attempt to conceive, Katie felt herself becoming more and more disheartened. Yet it wasn't until her third failed in vitro fertilization attempt that she slipped into a serious state of depression. Reluctant to discuss anything but her fertility treatment and dreams for a baby, Katie began to alienate her friends and family.

"I didn't care about anything but having a baby of my own, and I shut out everyone I cared about—even my husband. Finally, my mom and husband convinced me I should talk with a therapist, who helped me see that this was a life crisis—that I felt out of control not only with my life plan but with my body. The therapist talked with me about ways to cope with the stress and how to talk with my husband and friends about what I was experiencing. I felt supported and not so alone. I began to relax and take part in activities I used to enjoy, such as roller blading, traveling, and long dinners at my favorite restaurants. Now, although I'd still like to be a mother someday, I know I can be happy with or without a baby."

Overcoming Panic and Denial

At first, the mere thought of infertility sends most women trying to conceive into panic and denial. They push it out of their minds and take the advice of friends to relax, take a vacation, use an ovulation kit, even try sexual positions thought to increase the chance of pregnancy. Anything to avoid that word: infertile.

Denial is the mind's way of pushing away a reality because it is painful. In most cases, the denial eventually begins to fade into gradual acceptance of reality. However, if one does not work through the denial, there is a danger of getting stuck in this stage. Consequently, the inability to accept infertility may hinder one's initiative to seek treatment. Such delays may result in more problematic diagnoses and extensive treatments down the road. This scenario only increases the emotional distress.

Beginning treatment is usually a sign that a woman has accepted her diagnosis of infertility; however, it is not uncommon for the denial to recur now and then throughout treatment. The nagging question "What if I never have a child?" may be ever present in one's mind.

Learning about treatment possibilities usually alleviates some of the panic. Many patients find themselves fascinated by the miracle of conception and the many ways that doctors have found to artificially achieve it. The mind races with possibilities, and excitement and hope build. But, for all its excitement, this stage of discovery also makes us more vulnerable. Disappointments may begin to mount when the cause of the infertility is difficult to pin down and when cycle after cycle produces no positive outcome.

Dealing with Anger

Anger is commonly experienced by both women and men coping with infertility. Considering that human emotions are not tied to logic, individuals will often misdirect their anger. Sometimes the anger is directed at one's own body for not "working" properly. In other cases, the anger is directed at a partner or oneself for not wanting to start a family sooner, for postponing treatment, or for not seeing a specialist sooner. Often, the anger is directed at others—relatives or friends—who get pregnant and have children with seeming ease. Sometimes the anger is directed at God or some other higher force.

Overcoming Guilt

Guilt is another common feeling associated with infertility. In order to make some sense of why this is happening, couples or individuals frequently look to their past for a reason. Usually what they come up with is not actually a cause for their infertility. For example, a woman who is experiencing infertility may think it is the result of a past abortion. But the fact is, unless there were complications resulting in tubal or uterine scarring, it is unlikely that the abortion has anything to do with her present infertility. It is important to talk about guilty feelings with a skilled infertility counselor and work on addressing and healing these feelings.

Understanding Envy

News that a friend has "accidentally" become pregnant with her third child may set off feelings of envy in those undergoing treatment for infertility. It may become difficult to feel happy for friends and relatives expecting a baby. For some women, a seemingly innocent baby shower invitation can invoke feelings of sadness, panic, and guilt. Again, emotions are not logical, and experts say these feelings are normal; there is no reason to feel guilty about having them. It's important, however, to recognize them so that you can use some logic in choosing how to respond.

Dealing with Grief

As they move through the infertility experience, many couples feel like they are mourning. Infertility does indeed involve grieving. Couples grieve their sense of loss at having had no children. It is a difficult grief to handle. It is not like grieving over the loss of a loved one. It is like mourning a dream that hasn't come true. Even though it is elusive, the loss is very real.

Acceptance

Finally, after moving through the stages of denial, anger, and grief, one gradually accepts the reality of an infertility diagnosis. At this point, the options include accepting that ongoing infertility treatment is part of life for a while, that adoption should be explored, or that living without children does have its benefits. Acceptance can come at any time during treatment or after discontinuing treatment.

Regardless of the outcome of fertility treatment, the infertility experience remains with most patients throughout their lives. It is revisited each time the idea of trying to conceive comes to mind, and even through the experiences of friends enduring the same kinds of treatments. Like other chronic illnesses, infertility becomes part of the person who endures it. If dealt with openly and honestly, it can make an individual stronger and better prepared to deal with life's unexpected twists and turns.

Strategies for Coping

Stay Informed

Staying informed is an important coping strategy. As with any medical treatment, hope and fear make patients vulnerable. It is important to understand the medical care, to know what tests have been done and what still needs to be done or rechecked if there were abnormal or borderline results. Keeping a list of questions to ask the doctor and taking notes at appointments helps patients stay organized and on top of their care. Getting a second or third opinion is also common during the course of infertility treatment.

When we started talking about our infertility struggle with family and friends, it gave us a different perspective. We realized we really weren't the only couple in the world having problems getting pregnant.

Connie, 32, expecting twins Diagnosis: unexplained infertility

Personal empowerment is critical not only to good medical care but to confidence and character building. The more patients learn and read about their conditions, the more empowered they become, and the more confident they are in making decisions.

Lastly, infertility patients should be extra kind to themselves during treatment times—spoiling themselves with the likes of manicures, massages, hot fudge sundaes, or buying a new outfit they've been eyeing for weeks. The key is to do things to help you get through the treatment with the best possible attitude.

Keep the Problem in Perspective

Even though coping with infertility seems all-consuming, it is important to make an effort to carry on with other aspects of life. Talk with close friends and relatives during the most difficult phases of infertility treatment, but don't let the topic dominate all your interactions with others. This may be especially difficult for couples in their 20s and 30s. These young couples are often surrounded by friends who are pregnant and/or raising children. Conversations tend to center around pregnancy and child rearing, leaving the infertile couple feeling empty and inadequate.

First, I was in denial of my infertility because I had conceived easily with our first child. I have also had feelings of guilt, disappointment, frustration, and inadequacy.
Barb, 33
Diagnosis: secondary infertility and Asherman's Syndrome

Of course, carrying on with a routine lifestyle while undergoing infertility treatment is no easy task. Without even realizing it, many couples find themselves planning their lives around treatment cycles. Taking a trip may be impossible because it interferes with the monitoring of infertility drugs. Switching jobs right now is a bad idea because pregnancy is surely right around the corner.

Shortchanging other parts of life because of infertility treatments only results in self-directed anger and resentment. It is better to go on with life despite infertility—making the same decisions regardless of trying so hard to have a baby.

Avoid Settings That Are Painful to You

If attending a baby shower would increase the pain a woman feels, she shouldn't go. A friend will understand. Consider asking another friend or family member to pick up a gift and deliver it. If it is painful to shop for holiday gifts in stores where young families are present, consider other options. Order from a catalog or on-line. Give a gift certificate or savings bond as a new baby gift to avoid pain from shopping for newborn gifts or clothes. This is a time for women to be gentle with and protect themselves. Particularly during treatment times, patients must take care of their personal needs.

Plan Responses to Hurtful Questions

It's important to keep in mind that many friends and relatives do not know how to handle a friend or loved one's struggle with infertility. These friends and relatives, who may have small children of their own, may feel awkward and uncomfortable because they don't know what to say. Keep in mind that it is difficult for many outsiders to think of infertility as a health problem. To them, those undergoing treatment are not sick, and in fact look normal and healthy. Comments such as, "You both just need to relax and practice a little more," are common. These comments are hurtful because they leave the infertile couple feeling alone and misunderstood. Similarly, such questions as "When are you going to start a family?" seem innocent and appropriate for a couple who has been married several years. Yet to those experiencing infertility problems, these questions may feel like blows to the stomach.

One way to cope with such questions is to educate loved ones about the medical facts and to tell them how they can be most helpful. Help them understand that saying something as simple as, "I'm sorry you're going through this, what can I do to help?" can sustain and strengthen the relationship. Others may choose to quickly put the topic to rest by saying honestly, "We're trying and hope we're fortunate enough to have children one day." Others develop an answer they're comfortable with and use it again and again.

It is up to the couple to decide together how much detail they want to share with others and to gently let friends and relatives know that discussing the situation at every turn may be depressing—particularly if the news is not good. Sometimes that means friends and relatives simply need to be told that a change of subject— rather than a lengthy discussion—is the best prescription right now.

> *Before we had the girls, I felt frustrated, bitter, anxious, and very much a failure as a woman. Infertility was rough on my self-esteem. I lost a sense of control of my life's direction. Treatment can seem like a part-time job, and it can wear you down.*
> *Jeana, 37*
> *Diagnosis: hormonal imbalance, tubal factor, endometriosis, and unicorneate uterus*

Attend Support Groups

Although it is natural for a person to be initially hesitant about joining a support group, inclusion in such a group can be sanity-saving. Hearing other people's infertility stories helps us realize that we are not alone in our struggle. Communicating with others who are going through the same painful experience nourishes us emotionally and helps us find new ways of coping.

There are several national organizations that offer support groups and information for couples suffering from infertility. Perhaps one of the best known is RESOLVE, the National Infertility Association. The organization has local chapters in more than forty states. Also, International Infertility Council on Information Dissemination (INCIID) offers 140 on-line, interactive forums covering subjects from infertility and adoption to miscarriage and pregnancy after infertility. Another organization, the American Infertility Association (AIA), also offers information on how to find support groups. The Polycystic Ovarian Syndrome Association (PCOSA) offers information and support for women with PCOS. Information about these organizations is included in the Resource section at the back of this book.

Keep a Journal

Experts suggest keeping a journal of your experiences during treatment, taking special care to record your emotions. Journaling can be an effective way of expressing emotions. It can also help us realize how much progress we've made when we look back over past journal entries. Putting a focus on gratitude also helps to chase away the blues. Some women start a "gratitude journal," making entries that reflect the good things in their lives, things they are thankful for each day.

Minimizing Stress on the Marriage

Going through infertility treatment can take an emotional toll on a marriage. The woman must endure the strain of months, perhaps years, of treatments. At the same time, her husband may feel helpless watching her go through tests, shots, and procedures. He may feel removed from the process yet also feel the need to provide ongoing emotional support. Being unable to "fix" the problem for the woman he loves is frustrating to most men. Husbands often do not share the pain they are feeling over not having a child because they want to protect their wives.

Unfortunately, this can lead to feelings of distance between a couple, leaving the woman feeling like she is the only one who wants a child and the only one who is devastated that it isn't happening. The best scenario for both partners is to share their pain with each other. The commitment of each spouse to continued treatment is essential, as is open communication every step of the way.

When well-meaning people ask why we don't have more kids, I tell them we are undergoing fertility treatment and will hopefully have good news some day. I try to handle it in a positive way.
Kelly, 28
Diagnosis: secondary

Set Goals and Dates to Re-evaluate

Some couples find it helpful to follow timelines for re-evaluation of their treatment. For example, a couple may decide that if pregnancy does not occur within six months, they'll seriously discuss whether to continue treatment or pursue adoption.

Having a plan of action also may help lessen the urge to discuss the subject constantly. Experts suggest setting a time limit for discussing infertility, such as 20 minutes a day. Sit down for 20 minutes and discuss the current treatment options and each person's feelings about what is happening. Let each partner take 10 minutes to talk about his or her feelings as the other listens without interrupting. If one partner doesn't have enough to say, it's OK to hug or sit quietly together. When time is up, there is no more discussion until the next day. This way it doesn't come up over breakfast, lunch, dinner, and before bed. The idea is to guard against it taking over every facet of married life.

When to Seek Counseling

For some, ongoing infertility treatment can lead to severe, or clinical, depression. Individuals with severe depression are in need of a professional therapist who can help them through an intense emotional experience.

Signs of depression include:

- constant tearfulness, apathy
- loss of interest in favorite activities
- fatigue
- suicidal thoughts
- poor concentration and memory
- sleeplessness
- anxiety and inability to make decisions
- friends and family frequently asking what's wrong

Some women wait too long to seek help for depression. Much help, including the possible use of antidepressants, is available today. Of course, anyone with suicidal thoughts should talk with his or her doctor at once.

9

Multiple Births:
Risks and Realities

After just two rounds of injectable gonadotropins and artificial insemination, Tanya became pregnant. When an ultrasound showed three heartbeats, her joy was replaced by apprehension. She had read about the risks and hardships that accompany a higher-order (more than twins) multiple pregnancy and was aware that selective reduction was an option. After looking carefully at the risks on both sides, she and her husband decided to take their chances on the triplet pregnancy.

Tanya quit her job at 16 weeks gestation and was put on strict bed rest at 18 weeks. At 26 weeks, her contractions were escalating and she was admitted to the hospital for monitoring and intravenous drugs to hold off her labor. She delivered two girls and a boy at 30 weeks, all of them healthy and weighing in at just under three pounds. They spent six weeks in the neonatal intensive care unit, but eventually thrived.

Asked if she'd recommend a higher-order multiple pregnancy, Tanya responds, "Naturally, I love my children and feel blessed to have them, but I wouldn't wish the difficult pregnancy or exhausting demands of caring for three infants on my worst enemy. This isn't the preferred way to have children, and if I could have chosen to have them one at a time, I'd have jumped at the chance. Triplets are a lot more than just 'cute.'"

Multiple-Gestation Pregnancies

A *multiple-gestation pregnancy* is one in which two or more fetuses are present in the uterus. Some patients dread the possibility of having multiples, while others invite the opportunity in hopes that they will have more than one child and won't have to repeat fertility treatments. Regardless of one's view, it is important to remember that multiple-gestation pregnancies increase the risk of injury to mother and babies; such pregnancies are also considered the greatest potential hazard of medically assisted reproduction.

> *We hardly expected triplets. We were even less prepared to lose one of the babies. It was an emotional roller coaster, not knowing what to expect next.*
>
> *Julie, 34*
> *Diagnosis: hyperprolactinemia*

Multiple births seem relatively common today, but what are the risks of achieving a multiple-gestation pregnancy through infertility treatments? Overall, 39 percent of women using IVF have a multiple-gestation pregnancy. The statistics, from the Society for Reproductive Technology (SART), appear below.

Chances of Having a Multiple Pregnancy

With Fertility Treatment (With IVF)		**General Population**	
Twins	28 %	Twins	1-2 %
Triplets or more	11 %	Triplets	1 %

Contrary to popular belief, the risk of conceiving multiples is actually higher with ovulation-inducing drugs and intrauterine insemination than with IVF. Why? Ovulation induction gives physicians far less control over fertilization and consequent embryo development. With IVF, the patient and physician choose how many embryos to transfer to the uterus. Of those who do conceive twins, approximately one third will lose a twin in the first trimester. Of those who conceive higher-order multiples, approximately 50 percent will lose one or more during the first trimester.

Recommendations on Embryo Transfer

Concern over the risk of multiple births has been mounting in recent years. As result of this concern, a November 1999 study by the Centers for Disease Control and Prevention found that transferring three or more embryos in one IVF procedure needlessly increases the risk of multiple births without boosting the odds of achieving pregnancy in most patients. The study, which analyzed 35,000 IVF procedures, found that 42 percent of women under age 35 with numerous healthy-appearing eggs delivered a baby after IVF with one or two embryos. Using three embryos yielded the same success rate but boosted the percentage of multiple births from 20 percent to 40 percent of all deliveries. Multiple births increase the risk of injury to mother and babies and are considered the greatest potential hazard of medically assisted reproduction.

Currently there are no regulations guiding physicians in the decision of how many embryos to transfer to the uterus with IVF. However, the American Society for Reproductive Medicine now recommends that doctors transfer just two embryos (rather than three or more) when treating women under age 35 whose embryos appear robust. The Society also recommends each ART program keep their own statistics so they have a good grasp of their chances of ending up with a multiple gestation.

Some professionals are calling on physicians to work toward decreasing the number of higher-order multiple births by monitoring patients' cycles more closely and transferring fewer embryos during IVF. Yet, when balancing the cost of these procedures with their strong desire for children, some patients are still willing to take the risk of conceiving multiples in the belief it will help them achieve a pregnancy.

Selective Reduction

For those who conceive multiples and are concerned about the risks, *selective reduction* is an option. With this technique, the number of fetuses is reduced in order to increase the likelihood that the pregnancy will continue successfully. The procedure can be done as soon as multiples are identified on ultrasound, but usually before 12 weeks gestation.

I didn't think my pregnancy with twins would be high-risk. However, I spent six weeks on bed rest worrying constantly about my babies' being premature. I delivered early, at 34 ½ weeks. I am grateful that they are healthy and thriving.

Angie, 32, mother of twins conceived through IVF
Diagnosis: stage-three endometriosis

Selective reduction is accomplished by inserting a needle either through the abdomen or into the vagina and injecting potassium into the thorax of the fetus, causing the cessation of fetal heartbeat. This is usually performed by a perinatologist or high-risk pregnancy specialist. According to these specialists, the risk of losing the entire pregnancy from this procedure is about 15 percent. Other risks are bleeding, infection, and the leaking of embryonic fluid. Still, experts believe the procedure reduces further risks to the mother and the remaining fetus(es). It is recommended that the procedure be done when there are four or more fetuses in the uterus. Research also suggests that reduction of a triplet-gestation pregnancy decreases the risk to fetuses.

Choosing Selective Reduction

Of course, the decision of whether to undergo selective reduction is difficult for some patients to make. They have spent a lot of time and money trying to achieve a pregnancy. Then, once the pregnancy occurs, they are faced with the choice of whether to reduce the number of fetuses to a manageable level.

It is recommended that, prior to treatment, couples thoroughly explore with their physician whether they feel they could undergo selective reduction. Their feelings on this matter will influence the number of embryos to transfer with IVF.

IVF patients who are concerned about conceiving multiples can elect to have embryos stored and frozen for use in a future cycle. Although success rates are lower for frozen embryos, hundreds of babies are born this way every year. Similarly, a patient undergoing ovulation induction with intrauterine insemination can be proactive. If she has more than two follicles, she can opt to have those follicles *aspirated* (removed) and proceed with IVF or cancel the cycle prior to ovulation.

Sometimes, the decision about selective reduction is taken out of couples' hands when reduction happens naturally. In such cases, one or more of the fetuses will cease to grow and simply absorb into the others. This typically happens within the first trimester and usually causes no problems for the surviving fetus(es).

Opponents of selective reduction liken it to abortion, while proponents point to its life-giving qualities. Without it, higher-order multiples may die from a variety of pregnancy complications, including premature birth. In other words, twins will thrive much better in the womb than quadruplets, and will most likely be born a great deal healthier and later in the pregnancy as a result. The risks are high for higher-order multiples, but twins and even triplets often do well as long as they make it to at least 32 weeks gestation.

For couples having trouble making the decision after conception, professional counseling is highly recommended.

Risks for the Babies

All multiple-gestation pregnancies—including twin pregnancies— are high-risk, and the chance of complications increases with each additional fetus carried. Of greatest concern are the high rates of premature birth and the risk this carries for babies. Thirty to 50 percent of all twin pregnancies result in premature birth, while 75 to 100 percent of triplet births are premature.

The many risks of having premature babies include increased rates of cerebral palsy, mental retardation, vision and hearing problems, and chronic lung problems. Compared to singletons, twins are eight times more likely to have cerebral palsy; triplets are forty-seven times more likely to be born with it. Stillbirth and death during the first year of life occur in about

4 to 7 percent of twin pregnancies and 17 percent of triplet pregnancies.

And, even though the survival rates for premature babies are on the rise, survival doesn't guarantee normal development or good health. In fact, premature birth can have long-term effects on a child. A Canadian study published in February 2000 followed 150 premature babies into their teens and found that children born extremely prematurely—weighing two pounds or less at birth—experience significant learning difficulties that persist into their teenage years.

When I learned my wife was pregnant with triplets, I was both excited and worried. I thought about the financial implications as well as the toll it might take on my wife and our marriage.
Paul, 38
father of triplets

Risks for the Mother

Women who are carrying more than one baby are more likely to gain weight and grow larger earlier in the pregnancy than women carrying a singleton. They also tend to have increased morning sickness and become more easily fatigued.

But there are more serious risks as well. These mothers are at high risk of developing increased episodes of vaginal bleeding, detachment of the placenta *(placental abruption)*, preeclampsia, and postpartum bleeding. Also known as *toxemia*, *preeclampsia* is pregnancy-induced high blood pressure. If not treated, it can become *eclampsia*—a combination of high blood pressure and seizures. Eclampsia is a serious problem and a leading cause of maternal death; however, if proper treatment is provided, it is rare for eclampsia to develop.

Dealing with Complications

A preventive measure to lower the risk of many of these complications is strict bed rest—a state in which most women carrying higher-order multiples inevitably find themselves. Some women even require extended hospital stays for premature labor, with the average stay ranging from 2 to 12 weeks.

Bed rest may be prescribed for women who have early warning signs of premature labor, such as bleeding and cramping, or for women with high blood pressure. Some physicians recommend bed rest in the third trimester for any woman carrying triplets or other higher-order multiples. Usually, the woman can rest at home until intravenous (IV) medications or injections are necessary to control her contractions. Cesarean delivery is far more common in multiple births than single births.

Healthy Babies Still Bring Challenges

Despite the risks for complications, some women carrying multiples fare rather well with their babies. We have seen such celebrated cases in the media. Still, parents of higher-order multiples face many challenges after their children's births. As a result of pressures on finances and the difficult task of managing their babies' daily care, these parents have a divorce rate that is close to 70 percent higher than that of parents of singletons.

Resources are available to parents of multiples in the form of books, magazines, and organizations. Two notable examples are *Twins Magazine*, a national publication, and the Triplet Connection, a national organization that publishes a quarterly newsletter and offers a pregnancy information packet. Triplet Connection's pregnancy packet details the symptoms of and treatments for preterm labor; provides healthy diet information for triplet, quadruplet, and quintuplet pregnancies; and offers advice on coping with lengthy bed rest. See the Resource section at the back of this book for more information.

10

Pregnancy Loss

After trying to conceive for two years, Gina was finally pregnant after her first in vitro fertilization. Elated, she told a few close friends and family members. But when she went in for a blood test to check her hormone levels, her doctor found they weren't increasing the way they should.

Several blood tests later, Gina was told she had miscarried. "I was devastated. We had been through so much, and spent so much money, and it was all for nothing. I wanted to just crawl into my bed and stay there for days." Instead, she and her husband gave IVF another try, only to become pregnant and miscarry again. "I couldn't believe it happened again, the exact same way. Now I have a double fear: the fear of not getting pregnant and the fear of having another miscarriage."

Coping with Miscarriage

For couples who have had difficulty conceiving, pregnancy loss can be emotionally devastating. The excitement of the initial positive pregnancy test can quickly turn into a sense of failure and loss after miscarriage. Diminished hope of ever having a baby often accompanies these feelings, and many couples have difficulty finding the enthusiasm for continuing treatment. A short break from treatment is sometimes appropriate.

However, in most cases, pregnancy loss is not a reason to give up on conception. Miscarriage is not uncommon. It is estimated that one out of six of all human pregnancies ends in miscarriage, and 75 percent of these take place in the first 12 weeks of pregnancy. Two-thirds of miscarriages occur within two weeks after conception, usually before a woman even knows she is pregnant. Yet because those undergoing fertility treatment often discover the woman is pregnant very early on, they also suffer the emotional trauma that others may be spared.

With my first IVF cycle I became pregnant. I was due the same time as a co-worker. Then, I lost the baby at 8 weeks. It was painful to watch her carry her pregnancy to term. I would go into the restroom and cry and try to gather my strength.
Donna, 30
Diagnosis: tubal damage

It does appear that women coping with infertility do experience more early pregnancy losses than fertile women. In a 1995 study at Johns Hopkins University in Baltimore, Maryland, investigators tested 148 women for conception and early subclinical pregnancy loss—pregnancy and loss that occur without the woman's knowledge. Participants, two-thirds of whom were over age 30, provided urine specimens for more than 1,100 menstrual cycles. Women with signs of reduced fertility before or during the study had a 70 percent rate of pregnancy loss, with older women having a greater risk. This is compared with a 21 percent rate in women who did not experience fertility problems. The higher rate associated with impaired fertility did not change after administration of ovulation-inducing fertility drugs. The conclusion from the study is that women with fertility problems experience more early subclinical pregnancy losses whether or not they undergo fertility treatment. These findings also indicate that early subclinical pregnancy loss may be responsible, in part, for reduced fertility among older women.

Types of Pregnancy Losses

Miscarriages fall into several different categories. Note that the medical term for pregnancy loss before 20 weeks is *abortion*. Although it does not imply any intent to lose a baby, this terminology often sounds harsh to couples wanting a baby.

Pregnancy losses may fall into any of the following categories:

- *Blighted ovum*: A pregnancy that results in an abnormality in the embryo. The miscarriage shows up on an ultrasound as a dark, fluid-filled sac with no fetus.

- *Chemical pregnancy loss*: Occurs before a gestational sac forms, and the blood pregnancy levels do not double every two days as they should.

- *Clinical pregnancy loss*: Occurs after a fetal heartbeat has been documented on ultrasound.

- *Spontaneous abortion*: A pregnancy loss that occurs naturally, without medical intervention.

- *Complete abortion*: A loss in which all fetal tissue has been expelled from the uterus.

- *Incomplete abortion*: A loss in which some of the tissue from the pregnancy is left behind in the uterus, usually requiring a D&C (scraping of the uterine cavity).

- *Missed abortion*: The fetus has died in the uterus and has not been expelled.
- *Threatened miscarriage*: The cervix is still closed, but the woman is experiencing spotting or bleeding.
- *Inevitable miscarriage*: An open cervix with increased bright-red bleeding and cramping. Once the cervix is open, loss is usually inevitable.
- *Ectopic pregnancy*: A pregnancy that is lodged in the fallopian tube or other abnormal site.
- *Recurrent miscarriage* or *habitual aborter*: A term used when a woman has had three or more pregnancy losses.
- *Molar pregnancy*: An unusual condition characterized by placental tissue growing rapidly and causing high human gonadotropin (hCG) levels. Usually, no fetus is present in a molar pregnancy, only placenta. If a fetus is present, it is called a *partial mole*. Molar pregnancies occur in 1 out of 2,000 pregnancies.

Dilation and Curettage (D&C)

Whenever fetal tissue is left in the uterus after a miscarriage, *dilation and curettage (D&C)* is performed. This procedure involves scraping the uterine cavity of any remaining fetal tissue. It is usually done under general anesthesia and on an outpatient basis. If needed, the tissue then may be tested for chromosomal abnormalities.

Miscarriage: Causes and Treatments

The causes of miscarriage range from genetic and hormonal abnormalities to uterine factors and immunological problems. Even infections and environmental factors can play a part. Treatments vary with each diagnosis. Still, approximately half of all pregnancy losses go unexplained.

Age

The age of the woman when she conceives impacts miscarriage rates more than any other common factor. Women over age 40 have a significantly higher miscarriage rate; the rate of miscarriage at age 43 is 75 percent. This higher rate frequently results from random chromosomal changes that affect the ability of the embryo to develop normally.

Chromosomal Abnormality

One study found that 50 to 60 percent of all miscarriages in the first 12 weeks of pregnancy can be attributed to genetic or chromosomal abnormalities in the fetus. One type of chromosomal abnormality occurs when both parents have normal chromosomes, but these normal chromosomes don't link together or appropriately in the fetus. As a result, the baby ends up with abnormal chromosomes. Another type of abnormality occurs when one partner has a chromosomal abnormality and passes it on to the fetus. Tissue from the products of conception can be sent for analysis to ascertain if there was a genetic problem with the fetus. It is important to remember that both partners can be genetically normal and still have an abnormal fetus.

Unfortunately, only a costly chromosome analysis of each partner's blood (as much as $1,000 per person) can confirm a chromosomal abnormality. (Abnormal chromosomes in a partner account for only about 2 percent of miscarriages.) Genetic testing can also be done on the tissue from a miscarriage. But the test is unreliable because many times the genetic studies done on the tissue are contaminated with tissue from the mother. This testing does not always confirm an abnormal chromosome content and also costs approximately $1,000. The results usually take 10 to 14 days to obtain.

Abnormal Hormone Levels

Abnormal hormone levels are another common cause of miscarriage. One example is a deficiency in progesterone, the hormone that induces the development of the uterine lining. Without adequate progesterone, the lining will not develop sufficiently, and the embryo cannot implant and be nourished. This is called a *luteal phase deficiency.* The luteal phase is the second half of the menstrual cycle—the two weeks after ovulation—when the lining of the uterus readies itself for implantation of the embryo.

In some cases, doses of progesterone can be effective in creating a stable environment for the implanting embryo. Clomiphene (Clomid), given earlier in the follicular phase of the menstrual cycle, can enhance the production of ovarian hormones. This improves the development of the uterine lining and enhances progesterone production in the luteal phase.

Blood tests for progesterone levels in the luteal phase and in early pregnancy can determine if supplementation is needed.

Progesterone can be prescribed in the form of vaginal suppository, oral lozenge or pill, injectable oil, or vaginal gel (Crinone).

Women with endogenously high levels of LH are known to miscarry at higher rates than women with normal LH levels. LH suppressive medication may aid in preventing such pregnancy losses.

An overactive thyroid gland (hyperthyroidism) or an underactive thyroid gland (hypothyroidism) create another form of hormone abnormality. An underactive thyroid, or hypothyroidism, can severely impact a pregnancy in its early weeks, causing possible miscarriage. The precise cause for such a miscarriage is not known. Still, women with hypothyroidism who are pregnant should have thyroid tests done frequently in the first trimester.

> *I have had five miscarriages around 6 weeks gestation. I know it's not logical, but I find myself being resentful toward women who can conceive and carry babies to term with no effort.*
>
> *Robyn, 38*
> *Diagnosis: recurrent miscarriage*

Uterine Abnormalities

A woman with an abnormally shaped uterus may repeatedly miscarry. Approximately 10 to 15 percent of women with a history of recurrent miscarriage have an abnormal internal structure of the uterus. A *septate uterus* contains an excess wall of tissue (septum) that partially or totally divides the uterine cavity. Because the septum has poor circulation leading to poor lining development, a fertilized egg that tries to implant and grow there will likely fail. A *unicornate uterus* is shaped like the horn of a unicorn and is smaller than half the size of a normal uterus. An embryo would have difficulty implanting and growing in this environment. Problems also occur when a woman has a *bicornuate uterus*, which means the uterus has two protruding, horn-shaped cavities.

Pregnancy loss can also be the result of fibroids, or smooth muscle tumors, in the uterus. Such tumors may prevent the embryo from receiving an adequate blood supply after it has implanted. Also, scar tissue left in the uterus after an elective abortion, D&C, or from an *intrauterine device (IUD)* can make it difficult for an embryo to implant. This scarring condition is called *Asherman's syndrome*.

Most of these uterine abnormalities can be diagnosed by a hysterosalpingogram (HSG) or sonohysterosalpingogram (SSG). The HSG is an outpatient procedure done without an anesthetic. It involves injecting a dye into the uterus and looking for abnormalities on an X-ray. A sonohysterosalpingogram is an ultrasound performed while a saline solution is injected into the uterus via a small catheter through the cervix. Although not all uterine abnormalities require surgical repair, most can be corrected with surgery using a hysteroscope.

Incompetent Cervix

Another uterine abnormality, an *incompetent cervix*, means the cervical muscle itself is weak and cannot remain closed as the developing fetus grows. Miscarriages resulting from this problem typically occur in the second trimester, when the cervix painlessly dilates.

Sutures can be placed in the cervical tissue from 12 weeks gestation to prevent pregnancy loss. This procedure is known as a *cerclage*.

DES

In the 1950s and 60s, some women were prescribed *diethylstilbestrol (DES)*, a synthetic estrogen drug used to prevent miscarriage. Some of the children exposed to this drug in utero have either higher rates of cervical/vaginal cancer or some infertility due to abnormalities of the uterus. The most common abnormality is a small, T-shaped uterus. Other women may have tubal problems or irregular lining of the uterus. The miscarriage rate is higher in DES-exposed women, probably due to the fact that many of these women have uterine abnormalities that make it difficult for the uterus to stretch with a growing fetus.

Endometriosis

Women with endometriosis may be more likely to miscarry than women without the disease. Endometriosis may cause the ovaries to produce lower levels of hormones and poorer quality eggs, leading to increased likelihood of pregnancy loss.

Immune System Deficiency

The immune system also can play a role in miscarriage. A healthy immune system produces chemicals that aid in the formation of the placenta and blood vessels, structures that carry oxygen and nutrients to the baby. But immunologic problems can exist when the mother's immune system produces antibodies. Antibodies are normally protective—they're produced in response to the introduction of foreign material, such as bacteria, into the body. But in some cases they attack the body's own tissue, mistaking it for a foreign substance. These antibodies may indirectly cause clotting in the blood vessels leading to the developing fetus, depriving it of oxygen and nutrients.

Taking a baby aspirin each day throughout the pregnancy is one of the most common treatments for this syndrome. Acting as a mild anticoagulant, the aspirin is believed to stop the formation of the blood clots caused by the antibodies. Blood tests can determine if the antibodies are present.

Genetic Problems

Genetics do sometimes play a role in miscarriages. At least 50 to 60 percent of first-trimester miscarriages show evidence of genetic abnormalities. The most common genetic defect is an abnormal number of chromosomes. Again, genetic testing is complex and expensive, but many doctors recommend it after two or more consecutive miscarriages. If the placenta and/or fetus of a woman's first miscarriage has the normal number of chromosomes, her second pregnancy has only a 50 percent chance of being chromosomally abnormal. But if the first pregnancy is genetically abnormal, there is a greater chance that a second pregnancy will be abnormal. If a parent's chromosomes are abnormal, an increased chance of miscarriage is probable, although not all genetic abnormalities will lead to continued fetal loss. Genetic counseling is recommended.

Treatment options depend on the underlying problem and include continuing efforts for a normal pregnancy, pre-implantation diagnosis, or the use of donor eggs or sperm if either the man or the woman carries genetic abnormalities. Pre-implantation genetic screening of embryos before they are transferred to the uterus is now being done in some IVF clinics. A small tissue sample is taken from the fertilized embryo and studied prior to the transfer. The biopsy does not usually injure the embryo, and only the embryos that have normal chromosomes are transferred. Professional counselors are usually available to assist couples in making informed choices.

Environmental Toxins

In some cases, environmental toxins have been blamed for a miscarriage. Implicated toxins include glycol ethers, used in manufacturing and electronics industries. Another potentially harmful toxin is lead, found in paint, auto manufacturing, auto exhaust, batteries, and wood stains and varnish. Vinyl chloride, found in the plastics industry, furnishings, and apparel, is also considered potentially harmful.

Lifestyle Factors

Cigarettes, caffeine, alcohol consumption, and excessive exercise have been linked to pregnancy loss. Statistics show that women who smoke are more likely to miscarry than women who do not smoke. Nicotine causes the mother's veins and arteries to constrict. This decreases the flow of the blood that carries nutrients and oxygen to the growing fetus. Other studies show that two alcoholic drinks a day and more than two cups of coffee or three colas a day can increase a woman's chance of miscarriage. Combining cigarette smoking with alcohol and caffeine increases the risk.

Infection

Several infections can increase the risk of miscarriage. These include German measles (Rubella) and chlamydia. Any woman who is trying to get pregnant should be tested for German measles, and if she is not immune, she should be vaccinated with the live virus and wait three months before trying to conceive.

Another infection, *toxoplasmosis*, can affect fetal development that could result in a pregnancy loss or injury to a fetus. Women who are *first* exposed to the infection a few months before or during pregnancy are at risk for severe disease. The parasite that causes toxoplasmosis may be found in the soil in undercooked meats, and in cat feces. Cats which are allowed to go outdoors may eat infected mice or birds, passing the parasite in litter boxes. A woman could be exposed to the parasite while cleaning a litter box. To prevent toxoplasmosis, gloves are recommended for a pregnant woman when gardening, handling raw meats, or cleaning a litter box.

Warning Signs of Pregnancy Loss

Miscarriages are often, though not always, preceded by physical signs of pregnancy loss. Some women, especially those who do not experience any bleeding, are unaware of the loss until they are examined by a doctor. Still, vaginal spotting or bright-red bleeding are common indicators. Although bleeding does not necessarily mean a woman will miscarry, it's important to contact a doctor at the first sign of any bleeding. Other symptoms include cramping and clotting and a lack of pregnancy symptoms such as breast tenderness, nausea, and fatigue. In addition, lower abdominal pain on the left or right side may indicate an ectopic pregnancy.

Most importantly, a pregnant woman should never hesitate to call her doctor if she suspects her pregnancy is in trouble.

Coping Emotionally with Miscarriage

Feeling Misunderstood

Almost everyone knows someone who has suffered a miscarriage, but many couples are surprised at how deeply they feel their own loss. Most couples, and particularly women, feel an attachment to the growing fetus the moment they discover they are pregnant. Their hopes, dreams, and plans for a family are all wrapped up in this small being growing inside them. When the pregnancy fails to progress, so do their hopes, dreams, and plans.

This loss is often minimized by public misconceptions about miscarriage. Some women are told they didn't really lose anything because they were never really pregnant, especially in cases of a blighted ovum. Often, well-meaning friends or family members will say something like "Nature knows best." But for the couple who has had the elation of a positive pregnancy test and now has to deal with the end of that joy, this kind of remark brings no comfort. Friends often try to help by encouraging women to try again, never realizing their encouragement is discounting the would-be mother's sense of loss.

As the years went by, our families tired of seeing us trying to conceive, only to be disappointed. My mother berated me for spending time and money on treatments. She said, "If God wanted you to have kids, you would."

Jane, 40
Diagnosis: habitual aborter

Grieving the Loss

For these reasons, it is important that couples give themselves time to grieve and heal when miscarriage occurs. Couples often find it helpful to have some kind of ritual, whether it be planting a tree, buying a birdbath for their garden, or donating to their favorite charity in memory of the loss they have experienced. Having a ritual or commemorating the loss with something tangible helps make the loss feel more real. As with a death, it takes time to move through the process of grief and mourning. Society does not provide many structures for this particular kind of grief and loss, so it can be very difficult.

Discussing feelings with an understanding friend may help, as can avoiding the topic with those who don't understand. In some cases, a woman may even feel isolated from her partner, who may not share her same sense of loss.

If you find yourself in the following situations, it may be time to seek professional counseling:

- A persistent feeling of loneliness and isolation
- Inability to stop thinking about the loss
- Lack of people to talk to about the loss and related infertility
- Evidence that work and career are being affected
- A feeling that life is out of control
- Difficulty enjoying holidays and special occasions with family and friends

Once again, support organizations offer help to those couples coping with both pregnancy loss and infertility. In addition to providing the opportunity to meet others who have experienced similar losses, support groups provide tools for coping.

11

Ending Treatment

Mike and Sara had gone through four years of infertility treatment and tried nearly every available procedure before making the decision to end treatment. They both went through a grieving process for the children they would never have, and then they decided to look into adoption. Within two years, they adopted a baby girl.

Although Sara is very happy with her new family, her infertility experience remains a part of her life. "I spent four years in treatment for my infertility, and we never really found out why we couldn't have children. You don't forget an experience like that. But after we made the decision to stop treatment, I asked myself to define my true goal. I discovered my true goal was not necessarily to have a pregnancy, but to share my life with a child—to have a family, to be a mother. Mike and I are fully satisfied with our decision to adopt and wouldn't trade our wonderful daughter for anything in the world."

Making the Decision

For couples who don't take home a baby, ending infertility treatment can be the most difficult step of all. For some, this step happens during the treatment process. For example, some may stop after three failed artificial inseminations. For others, may stop after three failed artificial inseminations. For others, the decision to stop trying may come only after several years of treatment and many failed attempts to conceive.

Regardless of the timeline for ending treatment, for some couples it means giving up all hope of ever having a biological child. This decision often carries with it every emotion experienced throughout the infertility journey. Feelings of despair, failure, and grief are common. All these feelings are normal and a necessary part of healing.

When the doctor told me I probably would not conceive, it was like a slap in the face. I felt such a loss, like the death of a loved one. I mourned for months, then we decided on adoption. That was the beginning of my healing.
Cheryl, 37
Daignosis: scar tissue and polycystic ovary syndrome

Although some have extreme difficulty ending treatment, many couples report a sense of relief at having ended the ride on the "emotional roller coaster." After all, ending treatment also brings a new beginning. Some couples may begin the adoption process while others elect to live a child-free life.

Those who start their infertility treatment with a plan—and stick to it—usually have the easiest time making a decision to stop treatment.

When to Stop Treatment

Although the decision to stop treatment is a very personal one, it is important to be aware of signs that indicate the infertility treatment is having a negative impact on one's life. Asking these questions may help:

- Does debt prevent you from affording another cycle?

- Do you avoid being with friends because they "just don't understand"?
- Are you experiencing severe mood swings?
- Are fertility drugs causing you physical pain?
- Do you have sex with your partner only when you're trying to conceive?
- Is your infertility treatment interfering with all other aspects of your life, including your job and personal relationships? Are you showing signs of depression?
- Do you find you have less energy for medical appointments and less interest in medical treatments?
- Do you find yourself thinking more about being a parent than how to arrive at that goal?
- Is parenting more than pregnancy to you?

If either partner answers "yes" to many of these questions, it's time to evaluate the situation honestly and consider exploring options outside of infertility treatment. These include domestic and foreign adoption, surrogacy, and child-free living.

Before ending treatment, it's wise to consider getting a second medical opinion, if you haven't already done so. A second opinion may protect you from later wondering if you had tried every option possible or from thinking, "What if we had kept trying?"

Adoption

A wealth of literature is available on adoption, both domestic and foreign. Although domestic adoption has become laborious and difficult in recent years, it is still an option. The lucky ones get their names on selective agency lists or find babies through private attorneys—both costly avenues. Unfortunately for many would-be adoptive parents, the availability of U.S. babies is relatively low, due in part to an increased social acceptance of single parents and a steady rate of abortion. Some couples wait as long as five years on adoption agency lists. Also, the desire for open adoption on the part of birth parents has changed the landscape of domestic adoption. Open adoption permits the biological mother and often the father to be involved in choosing the adoptive parents. To varying degrees, the birth parents often stay in contact with the adoptive family.

I had a difficult time accepting that I could not get pregnant. Seeing pregnant women or baby commercials upset me. I had to overcome feelings of being a failure, of being defective.
Sheryl, 35, stopped treatment, planning to adopt
Diagnosis: endometriosis

Those uncomfortable with open adoption, or with waiting many years for a baby, may want to investigate foreign adoption. Although more expensive than domestic adoption due to travel expenses, foreign adoption is attracting more and more American couples and single individuals. Healthy babies are available in such countries as China, Korea, Russia, Romania, India, Guatemala, and the Philippines. Single women can adopt in China, and age restrictions are often looser than in the United States. The Chinese in particular are more open to older parents than are other foreign countries. In most cases parents must travel to the country for an average stay of two weeks to bring their child home.

Because children's pre-adoption care varies from country to country and orphanage to orphanage, it is critical to research agencies thoroughly and ask for personal referrals before proceeding with any adoption agency.

Child-Free Living

Not everyone wishes to consider adoption. Some couples feel they only want to parent a biological child. Others have fears about adoption or are uncomfortable with the expense of adopting; or they find the required home studies intrusive. A home study involves in-depth interviews with adoption officials, during which couples are asked questions about such things as their background, job, income, and extended family.

In the end, many individuals make a conscious choice to remain child-free. They focus on other life pleasures— building successful and fulfilling careers, traveling, nurturing relationships with friends and family, and pursuing personal interests. Many people channel their desire to be involved in a child's life by spending extra time with a niece or nephew, or by volunteering as a Big Brother/Big Sister or in a mentor program. There are many ways to touch a child's life without being that child's primary caregiver; virtually all children can benefit from the support and love of other adults in their lives.

Regardless of why a couple or individual chooses child-free living, it is not an easy choice to make, and the reminders are often constant and painful. Second-guessing after ending treatment is common: Did we make the right decision? Will we regret this someday? Yet those who decide to live their lives without children are not alone. More and more couples— including those without fertility problems—are making this choice every day.

Resources

RESOLVE

The National Infertility Association
1310 Broadway
Somerville, MA 02144
(617) 623-0744
www.resolve.org

RESOLVE's mission is to provide timely, compassionate support and information to people who are experiencing infertility and to increase awareness of infertility issues through public education and advocacy. The organization supports family building through a variety of methods, including appropriate medical treatment, adoption, surrogacy, and the choice of child-free living. Its Web site offers access to free publications on a variety of infertility topics. RESOLVE has chapters in more than forty states and has a physician referral system available. The organization's helpline hours: Monday-Friday, 9 am-12 pm & 1 pm-4 pm EST)

American Infertility Association (AIA)

666 5th Avenue
Suite 278
New York, NY 10103
(888) 917-3777
www.americaninfertility.org

The AIA is a resource for women and men needing reproductive information and support. Among the services the organization offers: a monthly newsletter, message board, live on-line chat, 24-hour helpline, support groups, information on libraries and resources, and physician referrals.

International Council on Infertility Information Dissemination (INCIID)

P.O. Box 6836
Arlington, VA 22206
(703) 379-9178
www.inciid.org

INCIID was created by three professional women facing infertility and pregnancy loss. Through their own experiences, INCIID founders identified a clear need for an easy-to-find, on-line resource of comprehensive, consumer-targeted infertility information that covered cutting-edge technologies and treatments. Since the founders' first telephone conference call in October 1994, during National Infertility Awareness Week, INCIID has grown into an international organization with members from every continent. INCIID stresses the importance of seeking early care with qualified practitioners, and outlines the criteria for moving to a specialist.

Polycystic Ovarian Syndrome Association (PCOSA)

P.O. Box 80517
Portland, OR 97280
(877) 775-PCOS
www.pcosupport.org

PCOSA seeks to promote awareness of PCOS and to serve as a support system with accurate information for women with this syndrome. Membership is open but primarily includes women who have either been diagnosed with or believe they might be diagnosed with PCOS.

American Society for Reproductive Medicine (ASRM)

(formerly the American Fertility Society)
1209 Montgomery Highway
Birmingham, AL 35216-2809
(205) 978-5000
www.asrm.org

This nonprofit organization is devoted to advancing knowledge and expertise in reproductive medicine and biology. Members must demonstrate the high ethical principles of the medical profession, evince an interest in reproductive medicine and biology, and adhere to the objectives of the Society. Its Web site offers a national listing of fertility specialists, ASRM publications on a variety of infertility topics, and a link to the ART Success Rates National Summary and Fertility Clinics Report.

Endometriosis Association

8585 North 76th Place
Milwaukee, WI 53223
(800) 992-3636 (in U.S.)
(800) 426-2363 (in Canada)
www.endometriosisassn.org

In-depth information on the puzzling disease endometriosis.

Fertility Research Foundation

877 Park Avenue
New York, NY 10021
(212) 744-5500
www.frfbaby.com

Established in 1964, this foundation is a comprehensive research and treatment facility. Its primary function is to diagnose infertility problems and provide treatment. Fertility counseling is also available. The staff includes specialists in gynecology, genetics, urology, sex therapy, endocrinology, immunology, radiology, bacteriology, pathology, and psychology. The foundation sees more than 2,000 patients annually.

CDC's Reproductive Health Information Source

4770 Buford Hwy NE
Mail Stop K20
Atlanta, GA 30341-3717
(770) 488-5372
www.cdc.gov/nccdphp/drh/art.htm

Offers assisted reproductive technology success rates reports, as well as information on the risks of conceiving and carrying multiple gestations.

Infertility Digest

Infertility Digest is an E-zine offering the latest infertility information and research. Articles cover fertility drugs, IVF, surrogates, and alternative treatments.

www.infertilitydigest.com

American College of Obstetricians and Gynecologists

409 12th Street SW P.O. Box 96920
Washington, D.C. 20090-6920
(202) 638-5577
www.acog.org

Comprised of more than 43,000 members, this group of professionals provides obstetric-gynecological care for women. The organization provides educational information to health professionals as well as to patients.

The Triplet Connection

P.O. Box 99571
Stockton, CA 95209
209-474-0885
www.tripletconnection.org

This organization provides a detailed pregnancy packet for mothers-to-be, covering such critical issues as nutrition, bed rest, and preterm labor. In addition, members receive a quarterly newsletter filled with stories and letters from other parents of triplets, quadruplets, and quintuplets.

Twins Magazine

5350 S. Roslyn Street, Suite 400
Greenwood Village, CO 80111-2125
303-290-8500
www.twinsmagazine.com

Published six times a year, this magazine covers all facets of parenting twins of all ages, with an ongoing column dedicated to parenting triplets as well.

Glossary

Adhesions: The union of adjacent organs by scar tissue.

Anovulation: Absence of ovulation, or monthly release of an egg, from the ovary.

Artificial insemination: Delivery of sperm to the woman's reproductive tract via a catheter.

Asherman's syndrome: Scar tissue left in the uterus after an elective abortion or D&C procedure, or from an IUD, which makes it difficult for an embryo to implant.

Assisted hatching: Performed on embryos before they are transferred to the uterus with in vitro fertilization, this procedure involves making a tiny opening in the zona, or outer wall, of the embryo using a laser or a special chemical to increase the likelihood of implantation.

Assisted reproductive technology (ART): A number of treatments in which eggs are removed from a woman's ovary, fertilized outside the body, and then transferred back into her body. The most common ART is in vitro fertilization (IVF).

Azoospermia: Absence of sperm.

Basal body temperature (BBT): Temperature of the body taken at rest. Theoretically, BBT rises after ovulation has occurred.

Bicornuate uterus: The uterus has two protruding, horn-shaped ridges.

Biopsy: Removal of a sample of tissue for diagnostic examination.

Blastocyst: The fertilized embryo after five days of development.

Blighted ovum: An abnormal pregnancy that results in a fluid-filled sac with no fetus.

Cerclage: Sutures placed in the cervical tissue to prevent pregnancy loss.

Cervix: Lowermost part of the uterus.

Cervical mucus: A lubricant secreted by the cervix that transports sperm through a canal in the lower part of the uterus so it can reach the fallopian tube and fertilize an egg.

Chlamydia: The most common sexually transmitted bacterial disease.

Chromosome: Threads of DNA in a cell's nucleus that transmit hereditary information.

Clomiphene (Clomid): The drug most commonly used to stimulate ovulation through release of gonadotropins from the pituitary gland.

Corpus luteum: Yellow mass in the ovary formed when the ovarian follicle has matured and released its egg. It secretes both estrogen and progesterone and sustains pregnancy until a placenta forms.

Cyst: Abnormal sac usually containing fluid or solid material.

DES (diethylstilbestrol): A drug that was prescribed to pregnant women in the 1950s and 60s. Some children exposed to this drug in utero have either higher rates of cancer of the cervix or vagina or some infertility due to abnormalities of the uterus.

Dilation and curettage (D&C): A surgical procedure that involves dilating the cervix and scraping out the lining of the uterus.

Donor insemination: Artificial insemination with donor sperm.

Ectopic pregnancy: Pregnancy located outside of the uterus, most often in the fallopian tube. Also referred to as tubal pregnancy.

Ejaculatory ducts: Male ducts that contract with orgasm to cause ejaculation.

Embryo: A fertilized egg.

Embryo transfer: Delivery of a laboratory-fertilized egg to the uterus.

Endometrial biopsy: Removal of a fragment of the lining of the uterus for study under the microscope.

Endometriosis: A disease that occurs when the cells that normally line the uterus implant in the abdominal cavity, ovaries, and around the fallopian tubes.

Endometrium: The tissue that lines the inside of the uterus.

Epididymis: The tightly coiled, thin-walled tube that moves sperm from the testicles to the vas deferens.

Epididymitis: Inflammation of the epididymis, which can cause scarring and blocked ducts.

Estradiol: The most active and naturally occurring estrogen.

Estrogen: The female sex hormone produced by the ovary that causes the development of the female characteristics and also plays a role in menstruation and pregnancy.

Fallopian tube: A tube located between the ovaries and the uterus that is responsible for delivering fertilized eggs to the uterus.

Fertilization: Joining of the sperm and egg to create an embryo.

Fibroids: Benign tumors found in the uterine muscle and connective tissue.

Fimbria: Fingered ends of the fallopian tube that pick up the egg following ovulation and send it down the tube.

Follicle: Cyst-like structure within the ovary that contains the immature egg.

Follicle-stimulating hormone (FSH): Secreted by the pituitary gland, this hormone causes the maturation an egg each month.

Gamete intrafallopian transfer (GIFT): A surgical procedure that involves placing both the sperm and egg directly into a woman's fallopian tubes.

Gonadotropin: A hormone that has a stimulating effect on the ovaries or testes.

Gonadotropin-releasing hormone (GnRH): A hormone responsible for helping to release (and monitor) the proper amounts of gonadotropins (FSH and LH) into the bloodstream.

Habitual abortion: Repeated miscarriages.

Higher-order multiple pregnancy: A pregnancy with three or more gestations.

Hormone: Produced by the endocrine glands, this substance travels through the bloodstream to specific organs where it exerts its effect.

Hostile mucus: Cervical mucus that impedes rather than aids a sperm's progression through the cervical canal.

Human chorionic gonadotropin (hCG): The hormone produced early in a pregnancy to help the corpus luteum produce progesterone. When given as an injection, it induces ovulation and progesterone production.

Human menopausal gonadotropin (hMG): The luteinizing and follicle-stimulating hormone recovered from the urine of postmenopausal women.

Hyperprolactinemia: Excessive prolactin in the blood.

Hypothalamus: The part of the brain responsible for maintaining body temperature, sleep, hunger, and reproduction. It also controls the hormones that regulate menstruation.

Hysterosalpingography (HSG): A test that involves injecting a radiopaque dye into a woman's uterus and tubes to visualize her upper reproductive tract.

Hysteroscopy: Procedure in which a tiny instrument is inserted into the vagina and up into the uterus, giving the physician a panoramic view of the uterine cavity and allowing the doctor to diagnose and treat or remove any uterine polyps.

Incompetent cervix: The cervical muscle itself is weak and cannot remain closed as the developing fetus grows.

Infertility: The inability to conceive after one year of well-timed, unprotected intercourse or the inability to carry a pregnancy to term delivery.

Intracytoplasmic sperm injection (ICSI): An assisted reproductive technology that involves injecting a single sperm directly into the center of the egg.

Intrauterine insemination (IUI): A procedure in which a very thin, flexible catheter carrying washed sperm is threaded through the cervix and into the uterus, where the sperm is delivered.

In vitro fertilization (IVF): An assisted reproductive technology that involves aspirating (removing) a woman's mature eggs, fertilizing them outside her body, and then transferring the embryos to her uterus for implantation.

Laparoscope: Fiber-optic scope inserted through the navel to view the reproductive organs.

Luteal phase: The second half of the menstrual cycle—the two weeks after ovulation—when the lining of the uterus readies itself for implantation of the embryo.

Luteinizing Hormone (LH): The hormone that facilitates the release of a mature egg from a follicle.

Macrophages: Activated cells that respond to foreign tissue or infection.

Male factor infertility: Infertility in the man's reproductive system.

Menopause: When menstruation has stopped for at least one year, usually around age 45 to 50, after which a woman is no longer able to become pregnant.

Menstrual cycle: The monthly cycle of hormone production and ovarian activity that either prepares the body for pregnancy or produces menses (the period). The cycle starts on day one of the period.

Miscarriage: Loss of a fetus.

Molar pregnancy: A pregnancy in which there is no fetus present, only placenta.

Multiple-gestation pregnancy: A pregnancy in which there is more than one fetus present in the uterus.

Oligo ovulation: Irregular ovulation.

Oocyte: Egg.

Ovaries: Two robin-egg-sized organs that produce the egg and female sex hormones.

Ovarian cyst: Noncancerous, fluid-filled sac located in or on the ovary that can be a normal component of the ovulatory cycle.

Ovarian failure: Complete loss of ovarian function.

Ovarian hyperstimulation: A complication that develops when the ovaries are overstimulated during the use of fertility medications. The ovaries enlarge and cause a buildup of fluid in the abdominal cavity. Symptoms include sudden weight gain, abdominal pain, nausea, vomiting, and low urine output.

Ovulation: The release of an egg from the ovary.

Partial zona dissection (PZD): Micromanipulation technique that creates an opening in the outer gelatinous coating of the embryo, which allows the sperm easier access to the cell membrane.

Pelvic inflammatory disease (PID): Inflammation and scarring of the pelvic region caused by untreated sexually transmitted diseases and pelvic infections.

Pituitary gland: A small gland within the brain that is responsible for regulating hormones associated with milk production and the menstrual cycle.

Placenta: An organ that develops within the uterus during pregnancy to provide the fetus with nourishment and eliminate waste products. It also produces hormones necessary to sustain the pregnancy.

Glossary

Polycystic ovary syndrome (PCOS): Hormonal imbalance that gets its name from the small cysts that form in the ovaries when a woman's ovulation process is not functioning correctly.

Polyps: Benign growths that can appear inside the uterus and can contribute to embryo implantation problems.

Preeclampsia: Pregnancy-induced high blood pressure. Also known as toxemia.

Premature ovarian failure: Loss of ovarian function before age 40.

Progesterone: A hormone produced by the corpus luteum in the ovary and the placenta (in pregnant women), it prepares the uterus for pregnancy and sustains that pregnancy.

Prostaglandins: Hormone-like substances released by the uterine lining that cause uterine contractions, resulting in menstruation.

Recurrent miscarriage: Having had three or more miscarriages.

Reproductive endocrinologist: A physician, an OB/GYN, who has completed a fellowship in reproductive endocrinology. This requires three years of postgraduate training in infertility.

Retrograde ejaculation: A condition in which semen is thrust backwards into the bladder rather than discharging from the penis upon ejaculation.

Secondary infertility: The inability to conceive after previously having carried a pregnancy to viability.

Selective reduction: Multi-embryo fetal pregnancy reduction performed to reduce pregnancy and prematurity risks.

Semen analysis: A test of the quality of the sperm, including count, movement, and shape.

Sonohysterosalpingogram: A procedure that involves using a salt-water solution during an ultrasound of the uterus.

Sperm count: The number of sperm in the ejaculate.

Sperm donation: Storage and use of an anonymous man's sperm with either an artificial insemination or IVF procedure.

Sperm motility: Motion of the sperm.

Sperm morphology: Sperm shape.

Subcutaneous: Under the skin.

Subzonal insertion (SUZI): A technique by which sperm are injected via a pipette through the zona (outer capsule of the egg) and are placed close to the cell membrane without actually penetrating it.

Surrogate: A woman who becomes artificially inseminated with a man's sperm and carries the pregnancy for an infertile person or couple.

Testicle: The male gonad, producer of sperm and male sex hormones.

Testicular biopsy: Procedure performed to determine if the cells that produce sperm in the testicles are present.

Testosterone: Male sex hormone responsible for the development of male characteristics.

Thyroid gland: Endocrine gland in front of the neck that produces hormones that regulate the body's metabolism.

Toxemia: Pregnancy-induced high blood pressure. Also known as preeclampsia.

Toxoplasmosis: An infection, caused by an organism found under-cooked meats, soil, and cat feces, that can affect fetal development and could cause a pregnancy loss.

Tubal ligation: Surgical sterilization of a woman by "tying" the fallopian tubes.

Tubal pregnancy: Pregnancy located outside the uterus, most often in the fallopian tube. Also referred to as ectopic pregnancy.

Ultrasound: Use of high-frequency sound waves to view internal reproductive organs.

Unexplained infertility: Diagnosis given when a couple is inexplicably unable to conceive.

Unicorn uterus: Uterus is shaped like the horn of a unicorn and is smaller than half the size of a normal uterus.

Urologist: A physician who specializes in the treatment of urinary tract and male reproductive disorders.

Uterine septum: An excess wall of tissue partially or totally dividing the uterine cavity.

Uterus: Organ in the pelvic region where the fertilized egg and fetus develops.

Varicocele: Varicose veins in the scrotum.

Vas deferens: The tubes through which sperm and testicular fluid move to the ejaculatory ducts.

Vasectomy: Surgical sterilization of a man by interrupting both vas deferens.

Zona pellucida: The protective coating surrounding the embryo.

Zygote: An egg that has been fertilized but has not yet begun to divide.

Zygote intrafallopian transfer (ZIFT): Procedure that involves fertilizing eggs in the laboratory and then inserting the resulting zygotes into a woman's fallopian tube.

Index

Index

About the Authors

Carolyn Maud Doherty, M.D., is board certified in obstetrics/gynecology and reproductive endocrinology. She is a member of the American Society for Reproductive Medicine, the Society of Reproductive Endocrinologists, and the Society for Reproductive Endocrinology and Infertility.

Dr. Doherty is a graduate of the University of South Dakota School of Medicine. She completed her residency in OB/GYN and also completed a fellowship in Reproductive Endocrinology at Rush-Presbyterian-St. Luke's Medical Center and Rush Medical College in Chicago, Illinois.

Dr. Doherty is in private practice at Nebraska Methodist Health System in Omaha, Nebraska. She and her husband, Michael Fee, have three children—Caitlin, Alexis, and Grant.

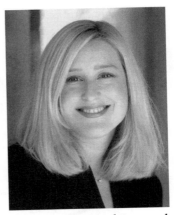

Melanie Morrissey Clark has been a writer and editor for more than fifteen years. She is co-author of the book *Straight Talk About Breast Cancer* (Addicus Books, 2002), and is Editor-in-Chief of *Today's Omaha Woman* magazine in Omaha, Nebraska. Ms. Clark holds a bachelor of science degree in journalism from the University of Nebraska; she lives in Omaha with her husband, Fred Clark, and their triplets—Cooper, Sophie, and Simon, who were conceived through in vitro fertilization.

Addicus Books Consumer Health Titles
www.AddicusBooks.com

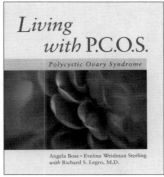